PRAISE FOR
EVICTING NAGATHA: A JOURNEY FROM SELF-SABOTAGE TO SELF-LOVE

"It's hard to be your best self when you keep getting in your own way. In *Evicting Nagatha: A Journey from Self-Sabotage to Self -Love*, the author does a beautiful job of helping us recognize that we cannot control others, we can only control ourselves. It will remind you of that hard teacher that no one wanted. Yet, when you got him you realized he was hard but because he was hard he made you better. He spoke the truth but loved you all the while doing it. That is what happens in *Nagatha*, you find that being truthful to yourself makes you better, all the while loving yourself through it. The first step in getting out of your own way is by evicting Nagatha. This beautifully written memoir will tell you how."

Nikki Stauffer
Healthcare
Professional Nashville, TN

"I am grateful to have read *Evicting Nagatha: A Journey from Self-Sabotage to Self-Love*, an identifiable Critical Parent Chokehold! It's a relief to see a step-by-step process designed for anyone to easily follow in an effort to expel this abusive voice once and for all!"

Cathy Resler
Hypnotherapist
Master Mental Health Counseling, Springfield College, Boston, MA

"I know Arvey personally and professionally, and she's without a doubt the most upbeat and motivational person to ever cross my path. If anyone can show us the way forward, it's her. Here's to letting Arvey set the stage so you can 'Flip Your Selfie' and 'Evict your Nagatha' once and for all. You'll be ever so glad you did!"

Carol Felzien
Vice President & CMO
Majestic Consulting Company

"I can think of dozens of women (and men) who regularly deal with these issues and will benefit greatly from this book. With the constant pressure from media and advertising to be perfect, drop-dead gorgeous, and always telling us how we can improve ourselves to be like the rich and famous, our true source of beauty and self-love is sabotaged. Finally, a book that offers an alternative pathway to happiness, away from the vicious pursuit of 'perfection'! Turns out - it's okay to be yourself. This incredible *no holes barred* book shows you how through real-life experiences and just the right touch of humor straight from Arvey's personal life."

Angelyn Garcia, B.A Journalism Emphasis
Certified Bible Health Counselor
Natural Health Counselor
Certified ProLiteracy Trainer

"Reading *Evicting Nagatha: A Journey from Self-Sabotage to Self-Love* has been truly enlightening and life changing. This is a great resource on how to take a step back from the pressure of society and reclaim our true beauty and self-worth. Arvey's ability to combine her personal experience with humor makes this book incredibly easy to relate to. I highly recommend it to everyone who struggles with self-sabotage and has been struggling to make the switch to self-love."

Laura Wilkinson
Professional Editor and Proofreader

"This book will make the perfect gift!" It is a gift that keeps on giving. It's a must-have. It's a LIFE-CHANGER!"

Tabatha Hale
Business Owner and Author, *Life's an Adventure*

"The book is full of insights that will help you change your life. Invest in yourself today!"

Cheryle Komnick
Business Founder, Owner & Operator Caloosa Tent & Rental, Business Influencer,
Board Member Pace Center for Girls and Greater Fort Myers Chamber

EVICTING NAGATHA

A JOURNEY FROM SELF-SABOTAGE TO SELF-LOVE

BY ARVEY KRISE

© Copyright 2023 Arvey Krise

Published by
EMME PUBLISHING LLC
Fort Myers, FL

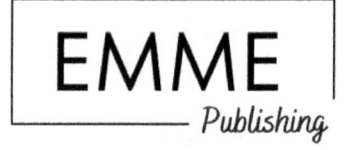

EMME
Publishing

ISBN: 979-8-9876264-1-2

All rights reserved. No part of this book may be copied or reproduced by any means manual, mechanical, or digital without written permission of the author.

*I dedicate this book to my biggest fan,
and the best roommate a girl could have,
My Husband, Randy.*

CONTENTS

I Want to Be Like Her 10

Introduction.. 14

Bar Carson Quote 19

PART I ABOUT YOUR ROOMMATE: Nagatha 21

Chapter 1: Worms 22

Chapter 2: You're Not Alone 32

Chapter 3: Meet Nagatha 40

Chaper 4: Where Does Nagatha Come From? 46

Chapter 5: Who Is Your Nagatha? 54

Chapter 6: Your Gatekeepers.. 64

PART II ABOUT WINNING: Nagatha Bootcamp............. 71

Chapter 7: Weaponizing and Winning 72

Chapter 8: People are Complicated..................................... 76

Chapter 9: Some People are Just Mean.............................. 86

Chapter 10: The Power of Your Critical Inner Voice....... 94

PART III ABOUT DISCERNING YOU: The Good Guy 105

Chapter 11: It's Always Been You.. 106

Chapter 12: Your Powerful Circle... 112

YPC DIAGRAM w ARROW... 117

YPC Blank Diagram 129

Chapter 13: You Can Change Your Brain........................... 130

Chapter 14: Why Do I Need to be Liked? 144

Chapter 15: It's Okay to Not Be Liked 158

Chapter 16: I Just Want to be One of the Guys 170

Chapter 17: Loving Yourself Isn't Good, It's GREAT 180

Chapter 18: The Many Faces of Nagatha 192

Chapter 19: Have You Met Your Ego? 202

Chapter 20: Do You Know Yourself? 214

Chapter 21: Why Do I Feel Lonely? 224

Chapter 22: Isolation Is Nagatha's Best Friend 238

Chapter 23: Friendship and NLMS 248

Chapter 24: Nagatha Nests 262

PART IV ABOUT EVICTING NAGATHA: The New You .. 269

I Am Confident Quote 271

Chapter 25: Conquering with Confidence 272

Chapter 26: Evicting Nagatha 282

Chapter 27: It's Been a Journey 292

Chapter 28: Happy Retirement Nagatha 300

Chapter 29: Finale: Dinner with a Friend 306

Chapter 30: Bouncers 308

Notes 312

I WANT TO BE LIKE HER

Today is the day.

She showered.

Carefully put on her makeup with precision. Not too much blush. Eyeliner crisp with just the right curves. Lip liner that gently accentuated and contained the stylish red lipstick.

Yes. Tasteful.

She slipped on her pale blue, freshly pressed size 6 vintage dress she had ordered from Amazon–a perfect fit over the petticoat that gave it just the right amount of lift. Red to accentuate the cascading flowers of her dress.

Her nails had been done the day before in the matching shade of gel and professionally shaped. Details mattered.

Next came the red open-toe sandals she buckled around her ankles. Awe, yes. Nothing makes a girl feel more feminine than high heels, especially red.

Misting the Chanel Coco Mademoiselle in the air, she glided through to capture the beautiful scent. Perfectly subtle. A trick she had learned long ago. It would never do for a lady to smell like cheap perfume.

Pearls. A single string around the neck with matching earrings. Class.

And then the grand finale. She donned the red *fascinator* that matched her shoes and the petticoat that graced the bottom of her dress–a must-have for a lady's tea.

As she looked into the tall mirror that had belonged to the sister-in-law of Thomas Alva Edison, a rare yard sale find, her lips broke into a satisfied smile as she twirled a bit, wondering if the original owner of the beautiful antique would be pleased.

Yes, today was the day. Her friend had invited her to be a guest at one of the two tables she reserved at the annual Grande Dame Tea–a *who's who* fund-raiser that honored three seasoned, esteemed ladies for their significant lifetime accomplishments that had impacted many lives in their wake. This wasn't her first, or even second time to attend this event. But she was hoping this time would be different. She was praying it would be the first time she would attend without the unwanted, uninvited accomplice.

Parking her car, she took a glance into the rear-view mirror, one final check, confirming that everything was perfect. Taking a deep breath, she confidently stepped out of the car and walked in full-stride, head high, to the front door. With a big, forced smile that wouldn't betray her, she opened the door of the venue. It was buzzing with excitement. The room was full of women in their dresses and hats, all dressed appropriately for a tea, many she had known for years, and all busy talking and laughing with each other in small groups.

Then the room went cold. Except for a few casual glances her way, nobody seemed to notice her. Nobody greeted her. But she looked so perfect for a tea, didn't she? The dress was right. The makeup, the fascinator, the shoes, the jewelry? And her big inviting smile. But it couldn't be any of those things... because with few exceptions, they hadn't even looked her way.

They hadn't seen her at all. She was painfully invisible.

As she walked through the room to the sign-in table, she continued to hold her head high and hold back tears... exuding confidence she didn't feel as she pursued her mission to fit in, offering friendly hellos to some who looked up briefly, reciprocating with a quick smile, feeling dismissed as none invited her into their conversation. This strong woman, the one who had it all together, who had been told by so many how they wished they could be like her, commanding a room, secure with so many friends, felt like she had been kicked in the stomach. Everything was wrong. She didn't belong here. Because nobody liked her.

This time wasn't different at all.

Then she knew.

She wasn't alone.

INTRODUCTION

Most of my life, I suffered...
Silently...
From "Nobody Likes Me Syndrome."
And the worst part?

I didn't even know what it was. Or that such a painful monster existed.

I just believed that people didn't like me.

And even more frightening... I thought I was the only one who felt that way.

The bottom line... I was *unlikeable*.

But sinking deeper and deeper into the depths of helplessness, I couldn't figure out why. Was I just so different from everyone else that I didn't know how to be like them or how to act?

I studied others. I struggled. I searched. I was lost.

For a born extrovert who loved people, loved to try new things, got involved with everything I could, and liked almost everyone, this was especially painful. I repeatedly analyzed what I was doing wrong that made people not like me. I was friendly... maybe too friendly, complimentary to others... maybe too complimentary, and went out of my way working hard... to be liked.

Maybe too hard.

My head reeled. Was I too loud, too forward, not forward enough, too happy, too sad, too intimidating, or dressing too weird? Just, too, too, too? I laid awake at night worrying if what I had said or done that day was stupid or offensive enough to make someone not like me. Tired and stressed from sleepless nights, I dreaded the thought of going anyplace where I had to face people. It was my kryptonite, my 'Achilles heel.' The harder it tried to bring me down, the harder I fought to beat it, albeit defenselessly. I had no knowledge or weapons. It made for a lot of miserable days of self-shame. I felt like I had been punched in the gut and all I wanted to do was isolate myself... safely at home.

Sound familiar?

Notice that in the first sentence I used the word suffered, as in past tense. After many years of suffering, beating myself up day after day, night after night... I'M OVER IT!

The better news... YOU CAN BE OVER IT TOO!

You can feel happy and love being around people, even groups of people. Why? Because after hours *and* hours of research, I discovered the secret. Which isn't a secret at all. Just hidden. It was there all along. I just wasn't seeing it. And it was so obvious... right there in front of me. I had to give myself permission to see it, and even more so, to believe it. It took knowledge coupled with understanding. One piece at a time. Or should I say, one "peace" at a time. A formula, a recipe for total peace and contentment. They say it's not what you know, but who you know. That's sometimes true, but to beat the "Nobody Likes Me Syndrome," it's what you know AND who you know... YOU.

I never believed I could beat the syndrome. And there's a reason for that–a reason many others share. You may not believe it either. Do you feel like I used to? Like you are different from others? Hopeless? Most people with "Nobody Likes Me Syndrome" do feel like this. How can you get over it when you are just not likable? Facts are facts, right? But I did get over it. And you will too, benefiting from not just my research, but from my *many* years of first-hand experience. I didn't just read about it, I *lived* it. My goal is for you to learn from my personal experience, which will enable you to live a happy and purposeful life. A life free of self-shame with no more searching for answers... a life of actually loving to be around others, and most importantly... you.

You were meant to be happy. To be the most you can be, where you want to be. Not someone you are ashamed of. I've been where you are. It hurts. When I started writing this book, I asked myself what I wanted to say to you. How I could help you get over the painful feeling of not being liked, and to be everything you can be... and are. The answer was to take you on the journey–my journey–of meeting the real you and clearly seeing others for who and what they are. They're not so bad. To go from being a desperate people-pleaser needing to be liked and loved by all... to accepting and loving yourself for who you are... just the way you are. No excuses. Ultimately, you will arrive at a long sought-after place of understanding and, even better, freedom, with an overwhelming awareness that perfect is overrated.

BOUNCERS

As you move through this book, you'll notice the bouncers at the beginning of some of the chapters. Think of them as ERASE and REPLACE. These are yours to tuck away for use when you need them. Have you ever been to a bar that has bouncers? They are hired to throw out unwanted troublemakers. The bad guys. You can probably name a few right now. Maybe they were kids in school, people at work, members of organizations, or maybe even so-called friends. When the voice in your head tells you something negative or hurtful about yourself... ERASE and REPLACE it with something positive. A bouncer. For example, in the chapter, Some People Are Just Mean, when the voice says, 'Why are you here, you don't fit in?' you erase that and replace it with, "*It takes grace to remain kind when people are cruel.*"

Nagatha is the troublemaker, the bully that lives in your head. She's an analogy that enables you to better understand the real culprit. Bouncers are your positive soundtracks, and they are there to throw out the troublemaker–to boot her out and stick up for you. Keep them close at hand because Nagatha will always try to find her way back in, looking for that vulnerable moment of weakness, the small crack in the door where she can sneak in. She's that latent urge for a cigarette in a reformed smoker when something stressful happens. But this time, it's different. This time, you're on to her and your bouncers will put her out on her ear.

But who is Nagatha?

She's a bad, uninvited tenant who is always causing trouble. But her lease is up... and you are not going to renew it. That apartment has a new and happy tenant who loves you... and you love her. She's your new best friend.

As you learn to understand yourself and other people, and as you become aware of who you are and what you want, your *team* of bouncers will grow.

Be warned. This is TOUGH LOVE, but it's nothing compared to what you've been putting yourself through with self-deprecating thoughts. You will be going through Nagatha Boot Camp, getting you in shape to fight and win this battle. The "Flip Your Selfie" actions will challenge and lead you to your destination–a peaceful and happy unapologetic YOU.

Before you go frantically looking through the Table of Contents for the "How to Do It in Ten Easy Steps" page, there isn't one. It's a process... one of learning, understanding, and conditioning with a lot of ohs and hmmms along the way that will subtly and suddenly add up without you being aware of it happening. It's work, but it's rewarding work. As you make your way through Nagatha, these moments of enlightenment will cultivate into a '*how did that happen?*' feeling like when you put a pan full of raw batter in the oven and, somehow, you magically get a beautiful cake in the end. And just like that cake, all you have to do is add the sweet icing and decorations on top... loving life and your new best friend... YOU.

Befriend this book. Get to know it. And you will be happy. Meet Nagatha... Your Critical Inner Voice... and take a journey to a better place. Don't forget to close the door and lock it on your way out!

(Tip: Nagatha could also be a Nagathon.)

> God gives everyone special gifts, but He also places challenges in our way to make us stronger. Some people meet these challenges head-on, right away, inspiring us all. Others take a "broken road," inspiring us all the more by overcoming not only external challenges, but perhaps the greatest obstacle of all—themselves."

Dr. Ben Carson, Sr. MD
Professor Emeritus of Neurosurgery
Johns Hopkins Children's Center
Excerpt from Forward of *What Are The Odds*
By Mike Lindell

PART I

ABOUT YOUR ROOMMATE: NAGATHA

1 WORMS

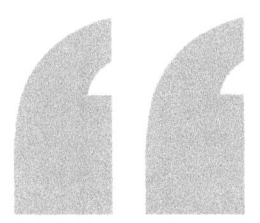

> When I was sixteen, nobody else talked like me. Nobody else sounded like me.
>
> -Linda Hunt

That woman you read about at the beginning of the book was me. Every word of it is true. In fact, just writing about it brought back all those painful feelings. Even though the room was full of women I knew, it took a lot of courage for me to walk into that social event. I didn't belong, and I was just embarrassing myself. It was obvious that nobody liked me!

But why?

PERCEPTIONS

A few years ago, while having coffee with a long-time dear friend, we started talking about perceptions and how others see us–a tedious conversation to be had only with someone you trust. It was an earnest heart-to-heart discussion between friends. Cheryl is a caring, practical business owner and knows the proverbial *everyone*. I valued her opinion. When she told me that everyone saw me as their friend, I was stunned. A friend? You could have knocked me over with a feather. It was a wonderful compliment, but I was genuinely surprised. As much as I have tried to be liked, memories of those long nights worrying about something I had done or said that *might* have alienated someone came rushing in. So, where were all of these people who, unlike me, saw me as their friend?

ARE YOU A THAT GIRL?

I'm often told I'm a *That* Girl–the one other girls look at and want to be like. Probably like many of you. The girl who is perceived by others as *having it all*–talented, beautiful, friendly, self-confident, sure of herself, secure enough to take on anything, not afraid of failure, funny, witty, self-disciplined, accomplished, educated, outgoing–AND has a secret she suffers from... "Nobody Likes Me Syndrome" (NLMS). If you knew me, you would be surprised. Even more shocking,

"Perceptions are reality at the time and can change on a dime."

- Arvey

many of the "I wanna be like her" women you regularly encounter battle this syndrome constantly. They are riddled with the twin demons of self-doubt and anxiety and are just as lonely in a room full of people as the wallflower in the corner. You may know one of them well, even look at her in the mirror. Women like us are perceived on the outside exactly the way we want to be by others. Whether you are a *that* girl or a *that* guy, the world is our stage.

Except for those of us who think we are the only ones with this terrible debilitating secret, nobody is aware of the ugly destructive monster we have lurking inside. But rest assured, we are not alone. Many famous people we love, admire, and fawn over and wish we could be like, including talented actresses, comedians, recording artists, and others, fight their own *Nobody Likes Me* demons, whether they are on stage or off stage. This might explain why their lives are train wrecks and they always search for more love and validation from others. But women are not the only lucky ones who struggle with this. Men share this battle too.

THERE'S NOTHING FUNNY ABOUT IT

Did you ever sing this little song with friends when you were a kid?

Nobody Likes Me
Everybody Hates Me
Guess I'll Go Eat Worms

Back then, we thought it was funny, skipping along and laughing with our schoolmates at recess, spitting out the word worms with a wrinkled-up nose as we sang this little jingle together. Great memories. But there comes a time when we realize there's NOTHING funny about it for many of us. There is probably not a *more painful feeling* in the world than *Nobody Likes Me*. Is there? If you live with this feeling, you know. You feel like your insides have been ripped apart. It's easy to fall prey to it, indulging in the self-shame, dwelling on feelings that lead to depression and loneliness. And for some, enduring sleepless nights like I did. It becomes reality in our minds. But that's where it is... in our minds. These feelings have no bearing on reality.

Like many of you, the episode of *Nobody Likes Me* at the social event I described earlier was one I routinely experienced in my life, starting when I was young.

I EVEN HATED MY HAIR

As far back as grade school, I remember hating my hair, my freckles, my clothes, and I was convinced that the other kids were talking about me behind my back. Maybe they were... because that's just what kids do. But some of us believed nobody liked us, and we were the only ones. We were too young and insecure to understand that kids can be especially cruel as their egos and superegos are developing and colliding with their ID. The triggers are endless. Those adolescent years were tough times for all of us trying to find our way–emotions raging, big ugly teeth looking for their place, figuring out who we were, and especially... where we fit in. Losing the vote for cheerleader or not making the basketball team could be brutal. And the last to be chosen by a side for dodgeball at recess was life-changing at the time. So, are those typical feelings we experience at that pivotal time in our lives something we grow out of? Or are they life-changing for some? Looking back on those sensitive and formative years, I can still feel the pangs from desperately wanting to be liked. For me, those pangs grew into a sledgehammer that didn't go away.

"NOBODY LIKES ME SYNDROME" ISN'T AN OCCASIONAL BAD DAY.

IT'S CHRONIC.

Starting at an early age, we all have 'those days' when we are not feeling the love. *"They don't like me. In fact, I don't like me."* Time to take a nap and start over. Even the most doted-on child will run and hide under the covers or strike out at their parents when they get upset and feel they aren't liked. Other kids aren't the only ones kids can be mean to.

"If you have never been hated by your child you have never been a parent."

—Actress Bette Davis

THE SYNDROME DOESN'T HAVE TO BE A LIFE SENTENCE

With an awareness and knowledge of:

- when these feelings start
- where our thoughts come from
- how our minds work
- why we think the things we do
- AND most importantly... who controls them...

the syndrome can become a thing of the past.

WHEN DO WE START CARING ABOUT BEING LIKED?

NLMS can lurk close by at an early age, but until we are mature enough for our conscience superego to become active and mediate with our ego to overtake our ID, we are not aware of our feelings about what others think of us. Our mental and emotional maturity dictate when that will happen.

Unless we develop a strong protective shield, hurtful thoughts about not being liked can become more self-destructive years later.

WHAT'S AN ID AND DO I CARE?

Dr. Sigmund Freud, the founder of psychoanalysis, defines our personality in these three parts:

ID - This is the primitive, or infantile, part of our personality that is the first to develop and controls our basic desires for satisfaction. For example, I'm hungry–NOW! It is all about me and its only mission is to get those needs satisfied as quickly as possible with no regard for others. The feelings of others are of no consequence or consideration in their demands. Think of it as the BRAT!

SUPEREGO - As we mature, our superego kicks in and we begin to develop morals and a conscience, which help us control our reactions to the BRAT, our ID. Developing morals and a conscience is what makes us aware of our feelings and what others think about us, eventually causing concern for being liked and approved of by others. The beginning of NLMS.

EGO - A deep and intricate subject that fittingly, as egos do, 'demands' further discussion. Why? To get over NLMS, a better understanding of the ego is imperative. While the ego is very confusing in psychology, we know it mediates or referees the demands of the ID (the BRAT) and the superego (the conscience), but the ego has many roles.

- It's the realistic part of the personality.
- It's the part of us that others see.
- Some professionals believe the EGO is your thoughts–good or bad. Some disagree.
- It's multifaceted and can be your best friend or your worst enemy.

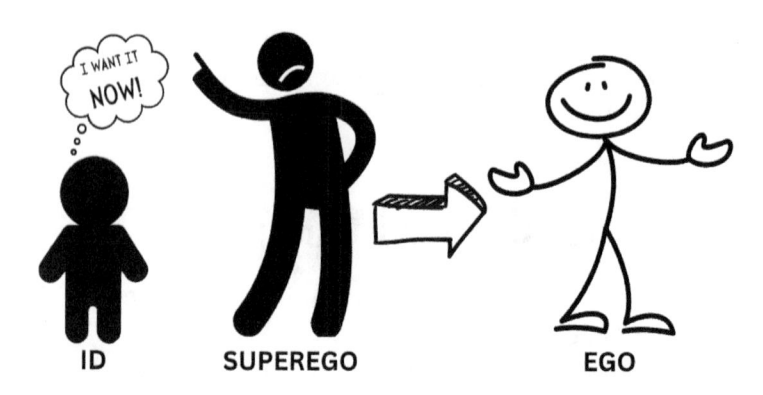

ID   SUPEREGO   EGO

YOUR CRITICAL INNER VOICE (CIV) AKA NAGATHA

All of you know how emotionally draining your CIV can be.

It constantly beats you up, judging everything you do:

- Comparing you to others.
- Reminding you that you are not good enough… or too good, but never right.
- Makes you feel alone and tricks you into believing… it's only you.

IF YOU LIVE WITH SELF-INCRIMINATING THOUGHTS LIKE THESE:

- *Nobody likes me.*
- *I'm not welcome here.*
- *I'll never get the job.*
- *They leave me out on purpose.*
- *Everyone has friends but me.*

ASK YOURSELF IF THESE THOUGHTS:

- *Keep you from achieving your goals.*
- *Make you feel bad about yourself or keep you awake at night.*
- *Disrupt your personal or social life.*
- *Cause you to avoid people, events, and social functions.*

You aren't destined to live like this. When you get the answers to the following questions in Nagatha Boot Camp (NBC), you won't have to!

- Is there a reason why people wouldn't like me?
- Is there a reason why I don't like myself?
- Do I do things that alienate people, making them avoid me?
- Why do I feel bad about myself, beat myself up, and even avoid social situations?

- Where do these painful feelings of nobody likes me come from?
- Why is it so important for me to be liked?
- Why can't I be liked by everybody?
- Why don't I have friends like other people do?
- Why am I so lonely?
- Do I isolate myself at the expense of being lonely to avoid the pain of NLMS?
- Am I the only one who feels this way?
- Where does this critical voice inside me come from?

And the one that matters most:

- How do I make it go away?

NOT by eating *Worms*.

THAT'S WHAT YOU'RE ABOUT TO FIND OUT

FLIP YOUR SELFIE ACTIONS:

Most of the above questions are rhetorical (at this point) and will be addressed in the following chapters. Start by doing a little self-discovery about your early years.

1. Take a trip down memory lane and think about how you felt about yourself in grade school and high school. Did you like yourself and who you were?

2. When do you remember caring about what others thought about you?

2
YOU'RE NOT ALONE

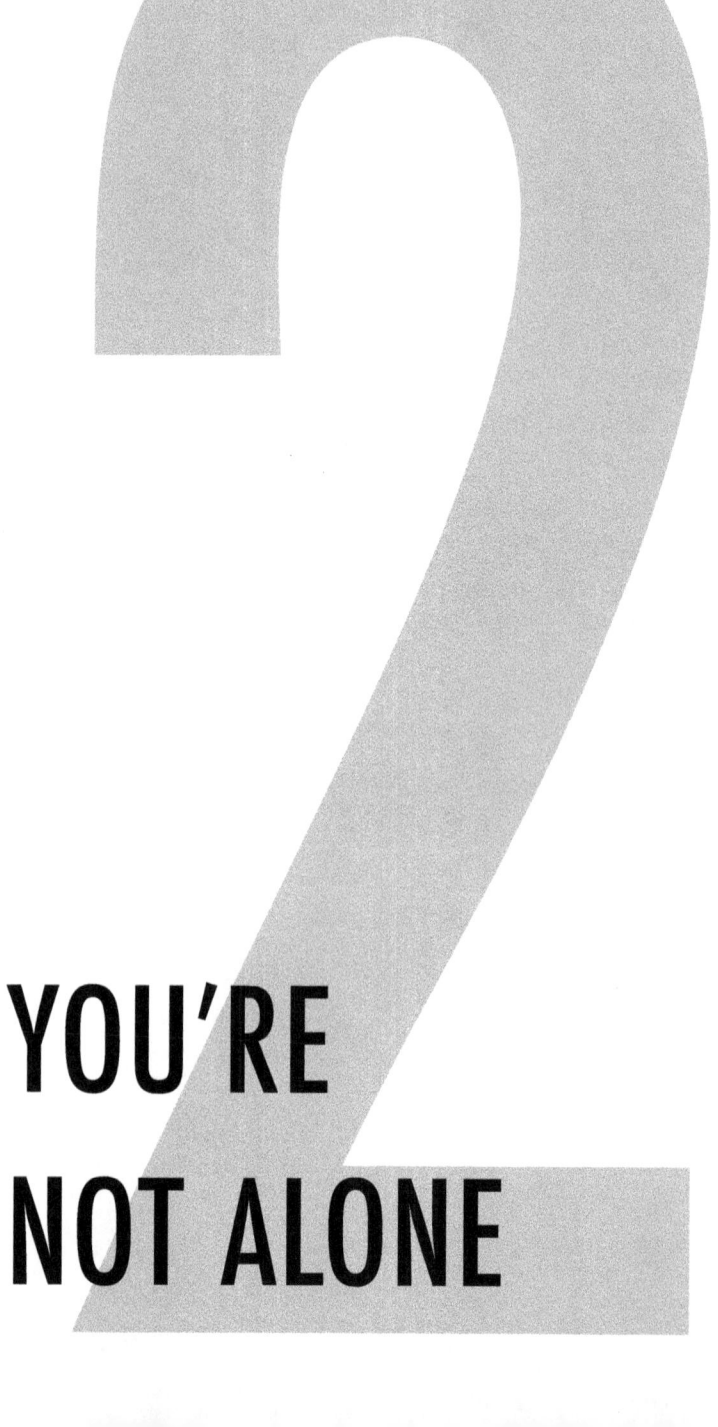

"

I want you to know that you are not alone in your being alone.

- Stephen Fry

"

BOUNCER:
I'm not alone, many others feel this way.

Why am I the only one who Nagatha picks on?
Where did that come from?
It's a *Nagatha-ism*.

She is hard at work. Always whispering in your ear, creating self-doubt.

While recently attending my granddaughter's dance competition in Orlando, a group of us were sitting around the pool having the usual 'where are you from and what do you do' small talk. A beautiful, classy woman with a huge, heartwarming smile and inviting personality was sitting next to me. She's someone you instantly like and who makes you feel like you just met a potential bestie. Like most people do when I tell them I'm an author, she asked me in her sweet Tennessee voice what I was writing. Maybe it was just small talk, or because statistically, 81 percent of people want to write a book. When I told her about Nagatha, the expression on her face changed. I saw it in her eyes and was not surprised when, with an *asking for a friend* expression, she asked, "When will it be finished?" I knew. Immediately. On the outside, she was a lovable, self-confident lady, but on the inside, she was a victim of NLMS. Sitting right next to me. If not for this conversation about Nagatha, her mask would have stayed securely in place, holding in her struggling self-esteem and the demons she lives with. Like many.

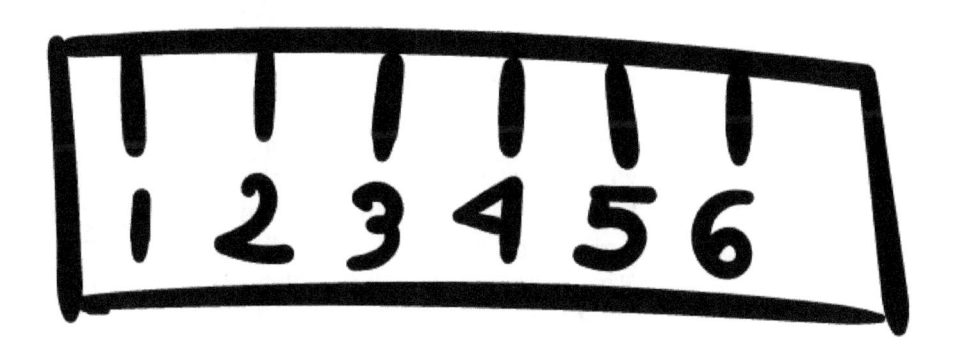

When psychologist, Lisa Firestone, conducted research using a scale measuring an individual's self-destructive thoughts, she found the most common critical thought people have about themselves is that they are different from other people. Human beings are a social species, and yet most of us feel on some level that not only are we different from others, but consequently, we are not liked. That puts us in the company of a staggering number of people we see and routinely interact with who privately feel the same way.

I used to think I was unique. Much to my disappointment, my Psych 101 instructor, Coach Duke, informed us one day that there is no such thing as a unique human experience. So much for feeling special. Isn't standing out as our own person a good thing?

WHY WE PUNISH OURSELVES FOR NOT BEING LIKE OTHERS

1. *We compare ourselves to others, wanting to be like them. But what makes them so much better than us? Not to mention the next crowd waiting around the corner? CUT... wardrobe change!*

2. Perception! We see what people want us to see. That next guy is struggling to fit in just like you. Remember the song, A Horse in Striped Pajamas? (Kaptain Kangaroo... don't tell me you don't remember). *If you put on striped PJs to be like that horse, you're not going to be anything like it when you take them off.*

3. Have you ever wanted so badly to be a part of the in-crowd but didn't know how? *They don't know either... they're just winging it. Unless they're leaders... try it! You be the in-crowd... but be warned: it's a temporary place.*

4. Negative environmental influences. Like in my day when parents were blaming the perils of today's kids on men wearing long hair and the singing and gyrating of that "godless" hellbound man, Elvis. *(They were out of control! Didn't Samson have long hair?)* You believe what you have pounded into your head over time.

5. And the biggest reason, our critical inner voice will never give us a break... no matter what we do.

The feeling of not being liked has been around for years. Even Charlie Brown in the Peanuts cartoon spouts with a sad face, *"I know nobody likes me."* Not only is it universal, but surprisingly, it's extremely common in extroverts as well as shy people.

THE TRUTH

You are more like other people than you think, boasting confidence *on the surface* while hiding b*ehind your mask*, worrying about what they think of you. But unless your knees are visibly buckling or you are running out the door with a pained expression, they are probably looking at you and wishing they could be *confident like you*. Instead of fighting their own pain, they keep safely hidden. Perception can be deceitful–a tool Nagatha uses to twist the truth and make you believe what she wants you to believe.

Although we can't explain why we would be an outcast, or be invisible, we still believe it's true. We analyze, agonize, and apologize, but it has nothing to do with *reality*! The misleading thoughts in our head shatter our self-confidence. We can't trust our perception of ourselves, much less those of others. It's like we are standing in a house of mirrors and using that distorted perspective to interpret how our actions are being judged and/or rejected by others.

You are probably asking yourself why we do this. We sound like an ogre in a fairy tale. But we're not in a fairy tale. This is a real-life nightmare. But you will wake up. The biblical expression in John 8:32 says the truth will set you free. As you discover more about *your* Nagatha, you will be set free of NLMS. She didn't get there overnight, so she won't go away overnight. It's a process. These are just the general studies. Think of the process like going to the beach and swimming in the ocean. To get to the big water, you have to wade over the broken seashells, and it is painful.

Nagatha can be your worst enemy, one you may not even know you had. Be it at home, meetings, work, restaurants, or sporting events, your CIV is always with you causing problems. Studies show it can even be responsible for *disease*... both physical and mental. Regardless of where you are... even with parents at a kid's dance competition, some people around you believe they are not liked and don't know why or what to do about it, but they drive themselves crazy trying. I was one of them for most of my life. It was a secret I was desperate to keep, afraid it would cause others to judge me. After all, it was my own *fault*... and I certainly wasn't going to tip others off by alerting them that I was an unlikeable person and making them look for reasons why. Now that I've evicted Nagatha, I know that nobody was looking for those reasons... except me. The nightmare was all in my head.

Is everyone going to like me? No, but that's okay. That just makes me one of the guys.

YES, YOU ARE DIFFERENT... IN YOUR OWN SPECIAL WAY. AND ISN'T THAT GREAT?

FLIP YOUR SELFIE ACTIONS:

1. 1. Do you feel you are different from other people?

    A. In a negative, *'I'm all alone'* way of thinking?

    B. In a positive, *'I want to be unique in who I am'* way of thinking?

2. How does that make you feel about yourself?

3. What would you like to change?

3
MEET NAGATHA

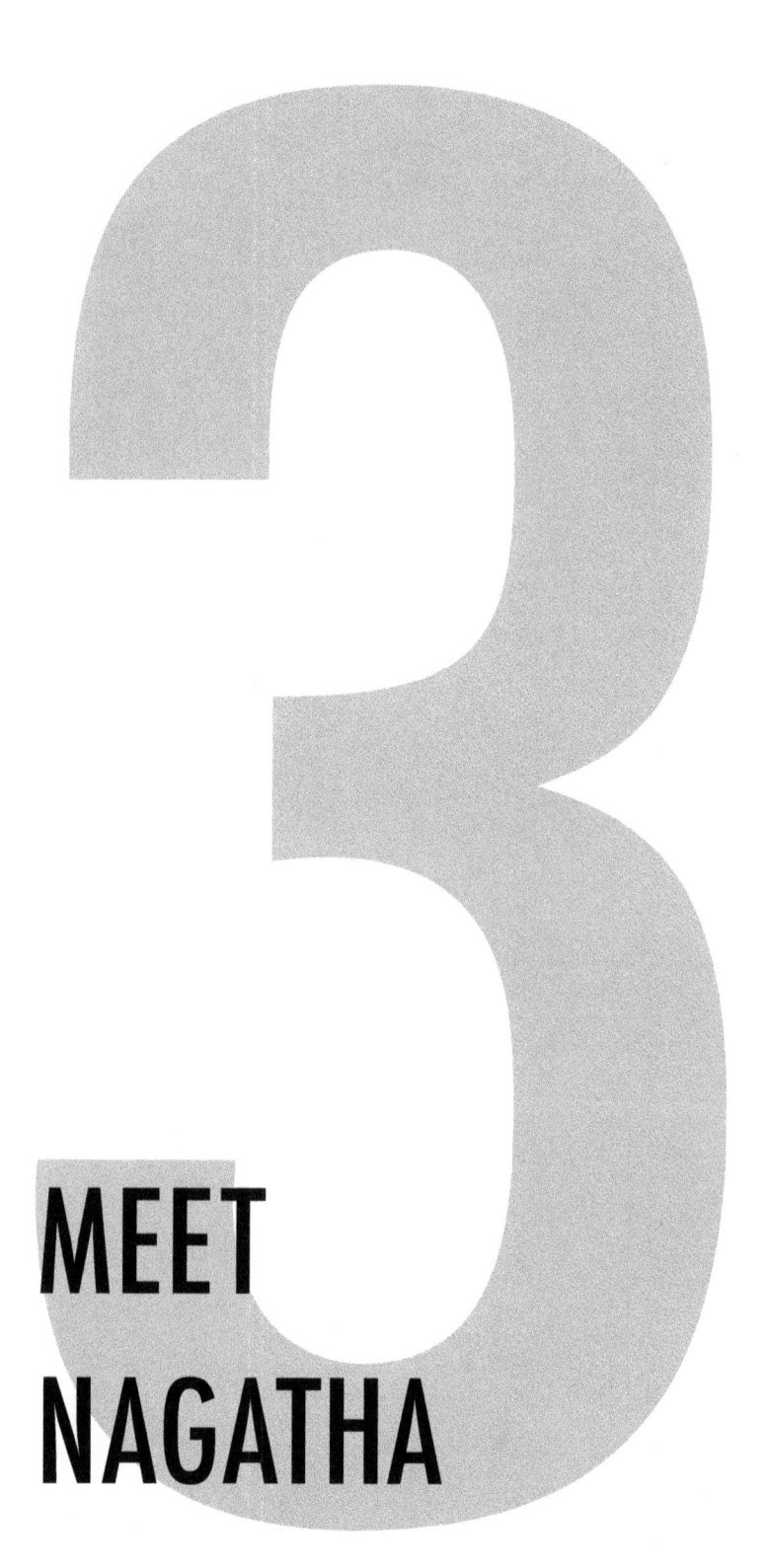

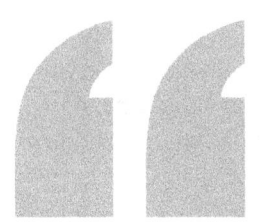

> Men are not prisoners of fate,
> but only prisoners of their own
> minds.
>
> - Franklin D. Roosevelt

You're right! You might as well face it. Nobody likes you. All the signs are there. You've alienated everyone. You're isolated and right where you should be. Alone. You don't have any friends. When you walk into a room, people purposely ignore you. You don't belong. People leave you out on purpose. Every time you open your mouth, you say something stupid. And worst of all, you are meant to be lonely. You even deserve it!

WHO SAYS?

Nagatha has moved in. She lives in the apartment upstairs and wants you to think she's your friend, looking out for you and telling you the way things really are, protecting you from the outside nasty world, or so she wants you to believe. Nagatha is real. Although you can't see her, she's a tangible being living side-by-side with the real you. She's your evil twin, who is not your friend. She's a parasite living off you, feeding off your weaknesses. At some point, while lurking and looking for a warm and cozy home, Nagatha found an open door, a way to creep in unnoticed and latch onto a vulnerable source.

AS LONG AS YOU GIVE HER ROOM AND BOARD... SHE'S NOT GOING ANYWHERE!

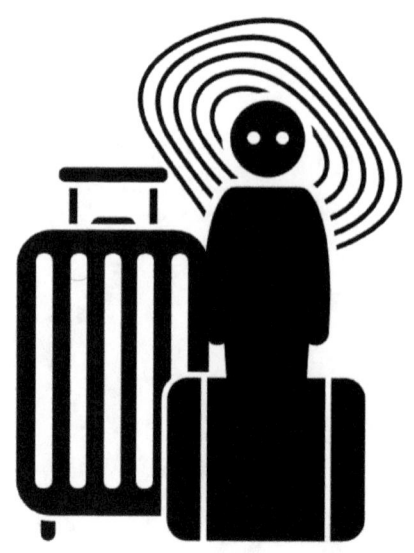

Nagatha is your nasty, critical inner voice who doesn't want you to be happy. She is a nag whose mission is to control you, dominate you, and keep you where she wants you. But she's very clever and good at hiding. She becomes such a highly subconscious and seamless part of your thought process that she's hard to recognize. You don't even know she's there, do you? She talks to you in your own voice and overrides all your positive thoughts. She's such a master at what she does that she can make you believe it's your own voice telling you all these horrible things about yourself... and even worse, you believe them. Her job is easy as long as you don't know she's there.

Nagatha wants you to wallow in self-pity. She knows how painful it is when she tells you things like:

- Did you notice how nobody said hello when you came in?
- Best to stay quiet. You're not even in their league.
- That group doesn't want you around. Did they even invite you to join them?
- You look ridiculous. Why would you wear that outfit?
- You deserve to be alone.
- You are fat and ugly and aren't worthy of being loved.
- Don't go. You'll only embarrass yourself. Stay home where you belong!

It's easy to develop a victim mentality, dwelling on feeling sorry for yourself, indulging in the low moments of dejection when Nagatha is constantly telling you that you don't deserve what you want because... you aren't good enough. Not to mention that horrible feeling that knocks the wind out of you. She confuses you with her self-shaming observations and purposefully misleading advice that makes you believe you are exactly what she says you are.

This voice can even make you afraid to socialize. You become so frozen with anxiety around people that you don't act like yourself, causing you to avoid situations where you would meet people and try to make friends. She wants you all to herself, hiding at home where you are safely tucked away in the arms of *your roommate*, who will protect you from yourself and all the people out there who *don't like you*. Even though you can't understand why. She is selfish. She tells you to stop trying because you are making a fool of yourself by ignoring all the signs that are *right in front of you*.

When someone doesn't make eye contact with you or look your way when you enter a room, she gladly points it out. "See?" she says. "They are wondering what you are doing here. After all, you don't add anything." When a friend doesn't text you back immediately, Nagatha is only too happy to explain. "They're obviously avoiding you. They're probably mad or just never did like you. You know they're with their other friends." So, you leave, feeling out of place... just like Nagatha said.

Nagatha's goal is to control you. By deeply wounding you, she causes you to shut down. This keeps you from functioning effectively and reaching your goals. She can fill you with self-doubt about everything you attempt and convince you to avoid even trying for fear of failure. She shreds your self-confidence, crippling you so badly with nerves that you can't even communicate effectively. Her never-ending, self-limiting advice and shame stifles you and leads you to a *self-fulfilling prophesy*. Nagatha is very good at what she does.

She actually lives in all of us. But she rears her ugly head more frequently and is louder and meaner in some than others. Nagatha understands your weaknesses, when you are at your worst, where and when to strike. She knows all your vulnerabilities and weak spots and is looking for times when you are more vulnerable than others to deliver a more effective punch. She knows that once we listen to her dangerous rhetoric that twists our reality, we can't trust our own perceptions about what others think about us.

But you can fight back by understanding the reasons behind what causes the self-destructive thoughts and insecurities you live with.

NOW YOU KNOW IT'S MORE THAN JUST FEELINGS. IT'S TANGIBLE AND REAL. IT'S NAGATHA.

In her book, *Yes, Please*, comedian, Amy Poehler, described this inner monster as "A demon voice." She wrote, "This very patient and determined demon shows up in your bedroom one day and refuses to leave. You are six or twelve or fifteen and you look in the mirror and you hear a voice so awful and mean that it takes your breath away. It tells you that you are fat and ugly and you don't deserve love. And the scary part is the demon is your own voice."

By the time Nagatha has convinced us we are worthless with all of her deceptions, we have lost touch with reality. We believe every negative thought about ourselves that she has repeatedly pounded into us, backed up with her misconstrued evidence, and there is no doubt in our minds they are true. The more we are convinced that we are losers, and the *so-called facts* that are right there in front of us apparently prove it, the harder it is to separate the truth from the lies.

YOU NEED THE FACTS
TO FIGHT AND WIN

- Who is Nagatha?
- Where did she come from?
- Who is my Nagatha?
- Am I alone?
- How do I evict her?

As the landlord, you need to understand that Nagatha is staying for as long as you provide her with the accommodations she needs to thrive and feed her with what keeps her alive, like any parasite. Once you know these things, you will be armed to evict her–for good.

4 WHERE DOES NAGATHA COME FROM?

> It is not what you say out of your mouth that determines your life, it's what you whisper to yourself that has the most power.
>
> - Robert Kiyosaki

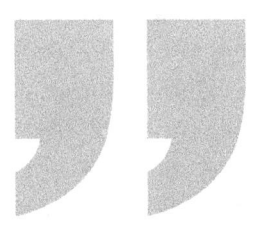

Once upon a time, there was a little girl who had some horribly unkind things happen to her in her short life. Consequently, these things made her a very unhappy child. They made her feel mean and ugly, and not like herself. She especially didn't like other people.

Even when she was a baby and made those cute little noises she had just discovered, nobody responded or showed her how much they loved her or her adorable sounds. She felt frustrated and empty. When she went to school, none of the other kids, or even her teacher, liked the things she said or did. They were mean to her. She didn't have any friends because she didn't know how to make them. Her whole life, she was terribly alone and depressed. Nobody knew how much she hurt inside, and the worst part... she didn't have anyone to tell.

One day at school, she went out to recess, and when she came back inside, there was a note on her desk. She was so excited that someone had thought about her. Maybe she did have a friend after all! But, when she read the note, it said, "You are the ugliest girl in school!" It was like someone had punched her. She was beyond sad and angry. The pain was unbearable. Cruel. Was she that ugly? Is that why nobody had ever responded to her new cute little sounds when she was a baby? Or why everyone was so mean to her? She was devastated, fighting back her tears. She just wanted to run home and hide, but there was no one there to make her feel better. They must have thought she was ugly, too.

To make herself feel better, she started telling the mean kids she didn't like them... and that nobody liked them. She called them stupid and told them everything they did was wrong and they should go home because they didn't belong there. She even told them they were fat and ugly. Doing this made her feel better about herself, like there were others like her, so she kept doing it until she got to be frightfully good at it! Before long, the only time she felt good was when she was being mean, criticizing and telling others how bad they were, and making them hurt like she did.

And so that's how she grew up to be.

One day, when she was all alone walking down the street looking for a place to live, she found a door that was cracked open. She quietly slipped inside and moved into the apartment upstairs. Nobody even knew she was there. But then she found someone to talk to who lived downstairs... someone who would make her happy again.

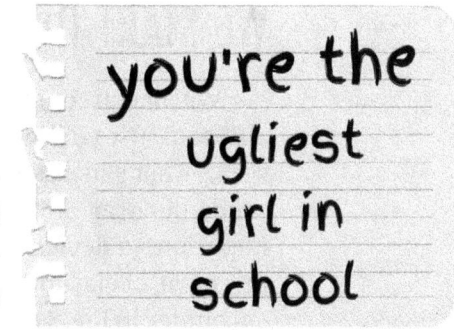

> you're the ugliest girl in school

Her name was Nagatha, and she loved her new home.

Dr. David Siddens, a clinical psychologist and colleague of mine during my nursing days, shared many stories with me that were a tremendous insight into understanding people, and the demons many secretly battle in their lives. Maybe he could see I was one of them. This is the story of the actual patient the fairy tale above was fabricated from.

An attractive middle-aged woman, who suffered from a terrible self-image that was deeply affecting her life, became a patient of Dr. Siddens. She fought serious depression, anxiety, and *Nobody Likes Me Syndrome* that affected relationships in her life, including her marriage. She progressively became more introverted and socially isolated. After hours and hours of exploring her life, nothing surfaced that could be attributed to her feelings of self-disgust. Finally, Dr. Siddens tried hypnotism, hoping that if she had been repressing something that would explain her low self-image, it would surface under hypnosis. And it worked. While hypnotized, she tearfully told a life-changing story that had happened to her when she was a little girl in grade school.

The class went to recess, and when they returned,
she found a note on her desk that said... you guessed it,
"You are the ugliest girl in school."
The child who left that note was Nagatha.

WE START OUT VULNERABLE

We all start out as innocent pieces of clay with a heart and soul just waiting to be molded into what we will become. That clay is soft and pliable–vulnerable to what life sends our way. During our early months and years, it is important to develop a protective outer shield around this raw piece of clay to protect us from the harsh elements we encounter in life. That shield is made of strong self-esteem and self-confidence and is the key to us becoming psychologically healthy. The stronger the shield, the more emotionally healthy and happy we will be.

WHERE DOES THAT SHIELD COME FROM?

Studies show that this protective shield starts to grow when a baby is born. It is formed when parents or caregivers make us feel our self-worth by cuddling us, mirroring our smiles, our cooing, and mimicking our noises and baby talk, all of which create feelings of acceptance and approval. Just this acknowledgment and adoration that caregivers show us throughout our infancy and on into childhood and adolescence, has a tremendously positive effect on our self-esteem and self-confidence, giving us a sense of belonging and validation. Hey, look at me, I'm one of the guys. This sense of belonging and being accepted is the protection that shields the vulnerable piece of clay we start out as from the storms we will encounter as we grow.

> **IMAGINE THIS VULNERABLE PIECE OF CLAY WITH NO PROTECTION, BATTERED DAY AFTER DAY BY THE STORMS OF LIFE.**

- Imagine the consequent bruises and scars that develop, resulting in undesirable defense mechanisms to guard and protect the soft clay inside.

- Imagine not consciously being aware of where the inner pain and wounds are coming from... and even worse, how to heal them.

How difficult it must be to start life without that shield of self-worth, having only basic physical needs met with no regard for emotional needs. Then having to first heal wounds from early battles you were not equipped to fight to enable you to start fresh from a level launching pad. But the great thing about self-esteem is that it is like an organ that can regenerate. Over time and under the right circumstances, self-esteem can be built (or rebuilt if necessary) and securely anchored to withstand the swells of life and successfully move forward and defeat Nagatha.

Our early encounter with caregivers is not only the first experience with our new world, it's our only experience. The first stroke of the brush on a blank canvas in a painting of our life. Are you wondering what parent wouldn't hover over their precious newborn and giggle, talk baby talk, and be enamored by their newborn's every move and sound? A parent with issues of their own. Or those who are products of their own upbringing. Sadly, what goes on behind closed doors can be shocking.

A good beginning is a solid platform... the first layer of the protective shield around that vulnerable, raw piece of clay. But life isn't always a fairy tale with a happily ever after, and having a secure, loving start does not guarantee that things will always be sunny without rain. Or thunderstorms and tornadoes. And throw in a few roaring high winds! Children who receive love and approval from the beginning of their lives get a strong send-off into the rest of their life, along with a springboard that can help them bounce back from pitfalls along the way. Having an initial dose of self-esteem can keep them anchored so they don't lose their balance and fly off in the wrong direction of insecurity... at least for a while. But at this early stage, it is still new and fragile.

> **"Children are like wet cement. Whatever falls on them makes an impression."**
>
> —Dr. Haim Ginott

The question is, where does Nagatha come from? She finds her way through a crack in the door when you are vulnerable. It could be after a single incident that left you exposed like the little girl in the story. Or perhaps from wounds that beat you down somewhere in your life, inflicted by a caregiver or multiple caregivers. Exposure to threats such as family violence, neglect, and controlling behavior are associated with higher levels of self-critical thoughts and emotions. A person criticized by parents for not performing according to their high expectations in school may develop a critical inner reel that repeatedly reminds them, "I am not good enough," or, "I am a disappointment." Sadly, one of the most painful experiences that can make you the most vulnerable to Nagatha is when someone you trusted to love and nurture you let you down by bruising you with their hurtful words or actions. Tragically, they are often someone who is hurting themselves, who used you in a misguided attempt to make them feel better about themselves. You were available.

Happens.

NOT YOUR FAULT. NOT YOUR FAULT. NOT YOUR FAULT.

Nagatha could have arrived at any time in your life when she found an opening in your back door... once you began caring what others think.

FLIP YOUR SELFIE ACTIONS:

1. Do you remember when your Nagatha arrived? Talk about it.

2. What was your response?

5
WHO IS YOUR NAGATHA?

> Listen to the Wind
> It talks
> Listen to the silence
> It speaks
> Listen to your heart
> It knows.
>
> - Buddha Groove

BOUNCER:
You're not a part of me. Why are you here?

❝ I know who my Nagatha is... my mother." These unsolicited words from a man I've worked with for years (while discussing cover ideas about Nagatha) came out of nowhere. Not trying to give moms a bad rap, but he immediately recognized the who of his critical inner voice. As he went into more detail about living with his Nagatha, his next question was, "When will this book be ready?" This is a question I get from many people as I watch their minds at work while describing the vastness of those affected by NLMS. Even unspoken, I see it on their face and in their eyes, and an occasional tear. Responding to their quiet with, "You want to know when it's going to be finished?" The answer is almost always... yes.

Sometimes it may seem like your uninvited demons never sleep or give you a moment of peace. They go on relentlessly with their same disparaging rhetoric. You know that catchy little annoying tune that gets stuck in your mind, playing over and over until you want to scream, "STOP!" And just when you think you have buried it with other thoughts or tunes, you realize it survived. It surfaces from the pile with... *I'm back and... you're still fat!* The people who write those jingles make a lot of money to annoy you for that reason! Bet you can finish this one... *give yourself a break today. So, get out and get away at* _____! Makes you crave a cheeseburger and fries!

But your soundtracks aren't about chocolate shakes or French fries. They are the consequences of hurtful experiences–a not-so-nice jingle that plays repeatedly and won't go away. They control your thoughts. Curious, isn't it, how you have to dig up the good memories, but the bad ones are always right there at the ready.

That's our Nagatha.

Who is behind the voice on your hurtful soundtrack?
Here's what you DO know so far.

- NLMS is a not-so-nice gift of your critical inner voice.

> **"Don't be a victim of negative self-talk. Remember YOU are listening."**
>
> —Bob Proctor

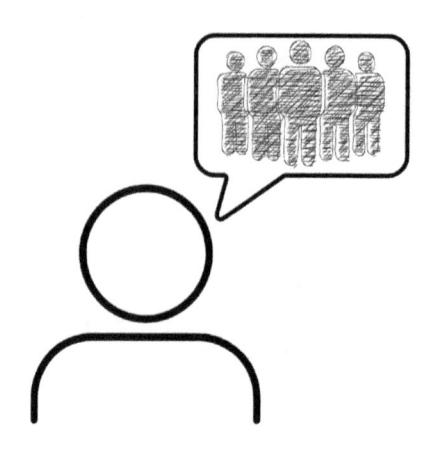

- It is not rooted in reality.
- Nagatha lives in us all.
- Its purpose is to maliciously demonize you.

We all have at least one voice lurking about; some of us have more... maybe a whole choir. But you're on your way to escorting them out of your head. Awareness is the first step that gets you halfway there. Just knowing there is a *legitimate* source of your self-punishing thoughts opens a new world of possibilities, questions for you to think about... and the power you possess to be in control. Possibilities that redirect you away from the road to self-destruction and put you on the road to understanding and *healing*. Just knowing you're not all those nasty things you've been made to believe about yourself... maybe most of your life... gives you hope. People do like you, and you do belong. The best part... you are about to turn your life around. As soon as you learn to believe it.

"WELL, HOW DO YOU KNOW THAT? YOU DON'T EVEN KNOW ME?" YOU SAY.

BECAUSE I WAS YOU AND I KNOW! AND YOU WILL TOO.

Knowing who you are fighting puts you on a level playing field with your nemesis. It turns uncertainty and fear into strength and confidence. You may already have a good idea whose voice is lecturing and criticizing you from its perch in your head, but you just haven't put 2 + 2 together. The mind is brilliant at suppressing what you don't *want* to see. It could be denying or repressing memories, preventing you from being conscious of it for its own reasons. There are documented cases of people developing alternate egos to hide from severe psychological pain they previously experienced. The mind is powerful and a great protector. If you don't know who your voice is, there's a good chance you will get some ideas as you progress through Nagatha Boot Camp and start listening. But don't be discouraged if you don't. Although helpful, it's not an absolute requirement to successfully evict it.

As you learn to know and accept yourself, you will crawl out from under it all to a new vista of enlightenment and freedom like you just opened your eyes for the first time.

IT'S A SENSITIVE SUBJECT

When researching NLMS, I did many confidential interviews with people from all walks of life trying to better understand who suffered from these feelings, why, and if they could identify their Nagatha. It was important to delve into what their childhoods were like, identify patterns and specific incidents that led to them, and how they and their lives were affected. Did their experiences lead to self-shaming, retreating, or even seeking isolation? And, if they overcame it, how? Hearing their *perception* of how severe their good or bad memories were revealed an interesting array of reactions on all fronts, with perception being the key component.

When I broached the subject, some people opened up immediately and talked freely about dysfunctional childhoods and how they resulted in them struggling with feelings of not being liked. Many people initially denied having negative thoughts about themselves. They smiled and acted astonished, telling me they never had them, they liked themselves just fine, or their childhood was wonderful. *Understandably, many people are private when it comes to sharing information about things that went on in their personal lives behind closed doors. Some are embarrassed and don't want to air their dirty laundry. They are also sensitive and **protective** of family members.*

However, by the end of our conversation, they became more comfortable. Nearly all of them talked openly about personal experiences they had growing up... *well, there was this one time...* and the negative effect on their self-worth.

Once that door was opened, it was like a relief valve went off. Very cathartic.

With some, the proverbial claws came out and they were visibly defensive before they realized this wasn't a personal attack. Not anymore. Pain from their past was safely tucked away.

Several admitted they had these feelings and were shocked in an almost healthy way when they discovered they were not the only ones. They were not alone.

A few said they had never had this happen, then after a little more discussion, admitted that *maybe sometimes* they did... a little.

What I discovered was that social status was not a determining factor. There are skeletons in every closet. Most families are *dysfunctional*, and this puts them on the normal side. That's life. Reality. Many still live with memories laced with pain... too caustic to bring to the surface.

Curiously, most of those who survived and successfully moved forward could identify their Nagatha. But not all, for their own reasons. Psychology is deep and twisted. While knowing is a start to defeating this monster, it may be too painful or frightening for some... hopefully, the time will come when they can face it head-on. For others, the pain may be buried too deep.

THERE IS A CONCEPT THAT PAIN IS MEMORY.

ACCUMULATED PAIN CREATES A NEGATIVE ENERGY FIELD THAT OCCUPIES YOUR MIND.

IT'S CALLED NAGATHA.

THE POWER OF IDENTIFYING YOUR NAGATHA

I read a story of a man who changed his outlook after a near-death experience. While hovering outside his body on the ground, he watched as they covered him with a sheet and loaded him on a stretcher before he was miraculously revived. Have you ever stepped outside of your feelings like an out-of-body experience, flipped your selfie, and *listened* to the critical voices in your head? Not just heard, but listened, as if you were listening to someone while enjoying a cup of coffee together. When you do, something enlightening may start to happen. Your mind will become more open to recognizing the voice as someone from your past, disguised as your own. Like my friend, who immediately identified the voice he had lived with most of his life when he heard about Nagatha. After accepting it as the *truth* for years, he suddenly saw it from a different perspective. We tend to see things in the now when what we are unknowingly experiencing is our past.

What happens when a memory surfaces and you know you recognize the voice?

It may be an emotional jolt like it was for me. But now, after experiencing life as a parent, I can look at things differently and it's easier to let it go. As if it was yesterday, I can still hear and feel the pain of things that were said to me when I was an adolescent, but looking at the whole picture now as an adult, I don't believe they were ever about me or meant to hurt me. I didn't deserve it, but I was also a hormonal, mouthy, sponge-adolescent living with my feelings on my sleeve, absorbing criticisms like a life sentence. Why? Maybe because the hormones were flowing, or I was without the protective shield I needed, or both. My parents were products of an unaffectionate childhood where words like love were not used. My dad grew up in a house full of boys and had preconceived ideas about his daughter, which influenced his parenting. That's not to minimize the things that were said. They were demeaning, insulting, and wrong, and I lived with those hurtful, negative self-perceptions for too long, not understanding where they were coming from but believing they were true. They caused me to not like me, and especially who and what I was. They made me miserable, feeling like I was unworthy of being liked.

Knowing changed that.

I want to be adamantly clear that discovering the identity of the voice isn't about finger-pointing, dredging up hurtful memories, or placing blame, regardless of the circumstances. You may be thinking, "But mine is much worse." *Regardless*, blame will change nothing. It only feeds the voices and keeps the pain alive.

MOVE OUT OF THE PAST AND INTO THE NOW

It's about healing... *empowering yourself* to rid your mind of the incriminating voices. Ask yourself this critical question. Do you want to heal? Or do you want to go on hating, which only hurts you? All our situations vary, and some are much worse than others. But they are behind you now, where they belong, and now is where you are. You have a choice of where you are today and will be tomorrow. Were your parents just being parents, maybe mimicking their own childhood and meaning no harm? Were you just being a kid, vulnerable to the fear of disapproval by those you needed to love you? By this time in your life, you may know firsthand that parents are people too. We are all products of our own childhood experiences... even parents. Now that my dad is gone, what saddens me more than the things he said is that I know he died hurting over it. He was a good man with some great parenting skills. Some were misdirected like we all have, but he loved me. Parents are just kids that grow up. Studies show that becoming a parent may revive bad feelings from your own past that you have to deal with.

Don't allow yourself to feel guilty about identifying the voices from your past that are the cause of your NLMS. It's therapy. And anger will only be the shackles that prevent you from moving on.

Remember the words of wisdom from my dad's best friend. *Youngin', "Your parents had parents, too. Forgiveness is the gate to freedom."*

The story about the little girl in grade school whose self-worth was shattered by a single note left on her desk by another child is an example of how Nagatha doesn't always come from someone at home. It can be anybody, anywhere. The stronger that protective shield, the harder it is to pierce, and the easier it is to recover from unavoidable blows throughout our lives.

Whatever your scenario is... *LET IT GO*. Send it back to where it came from... the past... close the door and step into now. I heard a preacher talk about a bird in a cage and how Satan kept banging away at that cage until, finally, the door of the cage flew open and the scared little bird flew away to freedom. Stop banging away at your cage. Open the door and watch the birds, the voices, fly away. Forever free. Forever gone.

Identifying the voice behind those lies allowed me to see them for what they were, like when Dorothy saw that the powerful Wizard wasn't powerful at all. He was just an insecure nothing preying on the weak to feed his own self-shame and feelings of inadequacy. Remember the change in Dorothy's self-confidence when she learned the truth. *Knowing is the real power.* It gave me the thumbs-up to see me–the likable me who is a good person–and the strength to be in control, to modify my behavior from negative to positive. The power of meeting me.

FLIP YOUR SELFIE ACTIONS:

1. Do you know who your Nagatha is?

2. What are some of the identifying factors, the words, phrases, and voice inflection?

3. If you haven't identified the person or incidents that are the source of your critical thoughts, ask yourself if you want to. Or are you in denial, afraid of what you might discover?

6
YOUR GATEKEEPERS

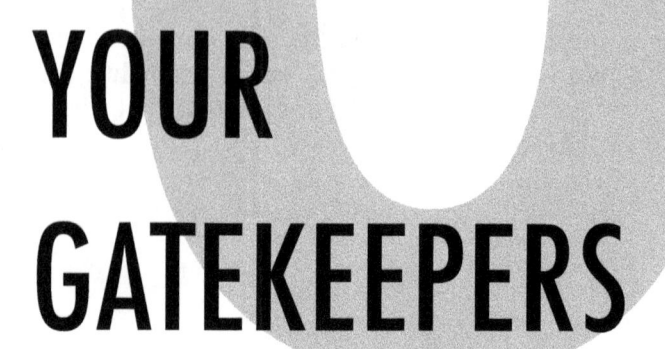

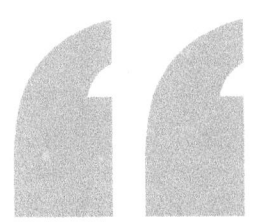

It is not the mountain we conquer, but ourselves.

- Sir Edmund Hillary

BOUNCER:
Being successful, being happy, and believing in myself are choices only I can make.

SELF-CONFIDENCE IS HOW CONFIDENT YOU ARE IN YOUR ABILITY AND SKILLS.

SELF-ESTEEM RELATES TO HOW YOU FEEL ABOUT YOURSELF.

BOTH ARE IMPORTANT TO OUR MENTAL HEALTH.

Why so much about self-esteem and self-confidence?

Because understanding and commanding self-esteem and self-confidence is your key to evicting Nagatha. While the two can support each other, they are not the same and you need both to be intact to be emotionally strong. They are your gatekeepers. They determine if you're going to have a good day or a bad day. They call the shots–make you strong or weak. They rule–putting you in control... or not.

Self-confidence is a result of your accomplishments, which gives you certainty about what you do and what you are capable of doing, while your self-esteem is a measurement of how much you like yourself. It's not uncommon to have one and not the other. In my days of NLMS, even though God had given me many talents I had honed and was confident in doing... much to the surprise of those who knew me, I didn't feel good about myself. My self-confidence left my self-esteem in the dust. Not liking myself demolished my self-esteem, which explains my need to over-compensate with high self-confidence. Knowing the difference is important.

***THEY CAN GIVE YOU COURAGE...
OR STEAL IT***

Self-confidence and self-esteem can even be a factor in how we wrongly perceive situations to be our fault when we are innocent victims, robbing us of the courage to stand up to ourselves... for ourselves and reality. As Nagatha convinces us with her punishing thoughts, *of course it's your fault,* we roll over to our low self-esteem. *I'm a loser, so I caused this to happen.*

Dousing ourselves with unfounded blame can have a devastating effect on us that can last for years, like when parents divorce or die, or we have other life-changing experiences or circumstances. It's especially prominent in domestic violence when the abuser, usually a victim themselves of self-hate, beats down the self-esteem of their victim so badly that they can make them believe they *deserve* to be beaten and even brought it on themselves. Another example is a conflict at work or with classmates at school that results in allowing and believing the mean words of others.

In the weakened state of low self-image paired with the fear of not being liked, it's easier to soak it up and take the blows, to deny our self-worth and our right to be who we are, than fight. It's all rolled up in the "Nobody Likes Me Syndrome" and is a result of how we see ourselves.

One of my close friends experienced tremendous issues with her self-worth when, at a sensitive and impressionable age, her parents suffered a serious, life-altering financial crisis. She abruptly went from being a secure child living affluently in a beautiful, large home, attending private schools, socializing with friends from successful families, and having parents who hosted lavish parties, to living in a small apartment in a less than desirable part of town and having to change schools and friends. In addition to the unexpected changes, she had to endure the toll the humiliation of hardship took on her parents' lives and marriage.

Her Nagatha convinced this angry, embarrassed little girl who was an innocent victim, to share the blame. Her self-esteem plummeted to rock bottom.

Case in point... because of the solid protective shield she developed as a child, years later, she worked through the an-

"It's okay to feel whatever you need to feel. Just promise me that you will never, ever feel guilty. Promise me that you will never blame yourself. It's not your fault."

—Colleen Hoover

> "Nagatha is painful memories in action."
> —Arvey

ger. Today, she has successfully moved on with her life and is a happy, successful adult who chose to learn from her painful experience. She now owns her self-worth, has a strong hold on her values, and firmly stands for what she believes in.

There will be situations in your life that can derail you... if you let them. How you react is directly influenced by both positive and negative experiences that left their mark on you. Without realizing it, you react in the way you have been programmed by your life experiences. It could be the hurtful way another kid reacted to something you did, a mean embarrassing prank, or an insulting remark made by a teacher or a parent. Or it could be positive interactions that catapult you through them with minimal damage.

Mike Lindell, founder of My Pillow and former drug addict, gambler, and alcoholic, shares potent words from Rafe Ronning in his book, *What Are The Odds - From Crack Addict to CEO*: "... the abuse of a child by an adult, particularly a parent, can produce a wound that a child doesn't even know is there." Ronning is a counselor Lindell interacted with at the Living Free rehab program at Living Word Church in North Brooklyn Park, MN. Lindell said, "Rafe talked about how these wounds can plant the seeds of addiction, which don't sprout until later, as that young man or woman begins to feel deep down that something is missing. That they are somehow odd or not good enough. That's when they start seeking ways to hide the pain." After Mike recovered from his addictions, he understood, through counseling, the impact of the sudden lifestyle change he experienced as a child. It doesn't have to be addiction. There are many undesirable ways our brains can find to try and mask pain.

If you hold out your hands with your palms up, like cups, and put all your glads in one and all your sads in the other, there will almost always be more glads than sads. It just seems that sads are heavier than glads because they are the ones that shatter your confidence. Nobody can ever have glads without sads, no matter who they are. That's life. It takes strong self-worth to look at yourself realistically and not take things personally, to own it when you are legitimately wrong, and to stand up for yourself when you aren't. It takes your security guards at their posts.

> **A PERSON WHO SUFFERS FROM LOW SELF-CONFIDENCE OR SELF-ESTEEM IS A MAGNET TO SELF-DEPRECATING PREDATORS.**

FLIP YOUR SELFIE ACTIONS:

I encourage you to think through your answers and write them down for your eyes only. You will be doing a more in-depth self-assessment in the chapter, Do You Know Yourself?

1. How do you feel about yourself and the person you are? Rate the strength of your self-esteem using a letter grade (A+ - F) and do the same for your self-confidence.

2. Think of a situation(s) where either your self-esteem and/or self-confidence has influenced the way you reacted. Write down how it affected your behavior.

3. Have you ever found yourself taking unfounded blame? Why?

4. Do you have the self-confidence to take a stand for yourself and the courage to accept responsibility when you are wrong?

5. Is your self-esteem as healthy as you want it to be? If not, write a plan to get it there.

PART II

ABOUT WINNING: NAGATHA BOOT CAMP

7

WEAPONIZING AND WINNING

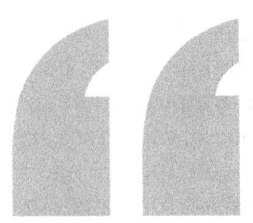

There is something I do not
know, the knowing of which
could change everything.

- Werner Erhard

For years, I fought chronic episodes of feeling sick. Weeks at a time, I was fatigued and dizzy, my head felt stuffed with cotton, and the symptoms left me weak, shaky, and even bedridden. Of course, we nurses are notorious for self-diagnosing, so I was convinced I had a terminal... something. It was especially scary for a high-energy, I can conquer the world in three easy steps kind of girl like me. Each time I seemed to recover from an episode and ventured out, in a few days, I was sick again. The pattern continued. Not only was I worried, but I was also mentally, emotionally, and physically exhausted. When one of my best friends called me sickly, I erupted. "I am NOT sickly and that's pretty rude," I said, only half believing it. But she was right. I was sickly. I just didn't know why. Nor did I know what to do about it.

Finally, I swallowed my I'm a nurse pride and saw a new doctor who ran a series of tests that involved a million tiny needles. The diagnosis was environmental allergies. That explained the on-off cycles. Relieved to find it was something I could defeat and win, I immediately learned what I could about allergies, how to fight them, where they come from, how they attack, and how to stop them. Soon, I felt strong and healthy and thanked my friend for opening my eyes to the facts.

Ignorance was my biggest hurdle. How could I fight something when I wasn't even aware it existed? Armed with this new knowledge, I was able to defeat this longtime enemy and get rid of the symptoms, becoming mentally, emotionally, and physically fit again... and WIN!

KNOW-ING IS NO-ING – A POWERFUL WEAPON

We know Nagatha's mission is to cause you misery by filling your head with self-destructive thoughts. This calls for a strategy. A plan. The goal is to not only kick her out, but to keep her from coming back. The way to do that is by filling the vacancy with a mentally and emotionally healthy tenant. You.

In Nagatha Boot Camp, you are going to get a workout that will get you in great shape to win mentally and emotionally. Building a strong, healthy mind will prepare you to win the battle. Just like when I was suffering without knowing the cause, until you have a clear understanding of what you are battling, you can't formulate a strategic plan to win. Knowledge is your first line of defense... and offense. A general would never lead his troops onto the battlefield without a plan to assure victory, which includes knowing who the enemy is, where they are hiding, how they attack, and the strengths and weaknesses of both his enemy and his soldiers.

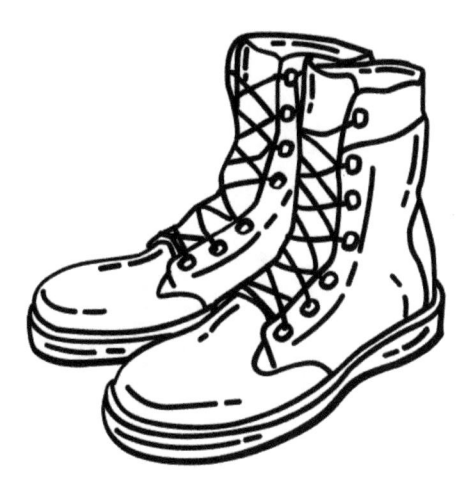

The goal of this training is for you to discover and understand:

- The frightening truth about your enemy
- People, including you
- The mystery of Being Liked
- Weaknesses and vulnerabilities
- Misperceptions
- Who's in control
- Isolation and loneliness
- Friendship
- Your Powerful Circle and ROI
- Bouncers
- Your new best friend
- Giving Nagatha the Boot

This is a journey that requires work and practice. You are not alone. Many are on it with you.

It starts with small steps of introspection and understanding along the way. You will experience a new awakening when you reach your destination and unlock the door to your new sense of freedom and joy. The boundless energy of just being you will put a bounce in your step and give you the confidence to see the world through distinct eyes. Yours.

THE MOST IMPORTANT WEAPON YOU HAVE IN YOUR ARSENAL IS YOU

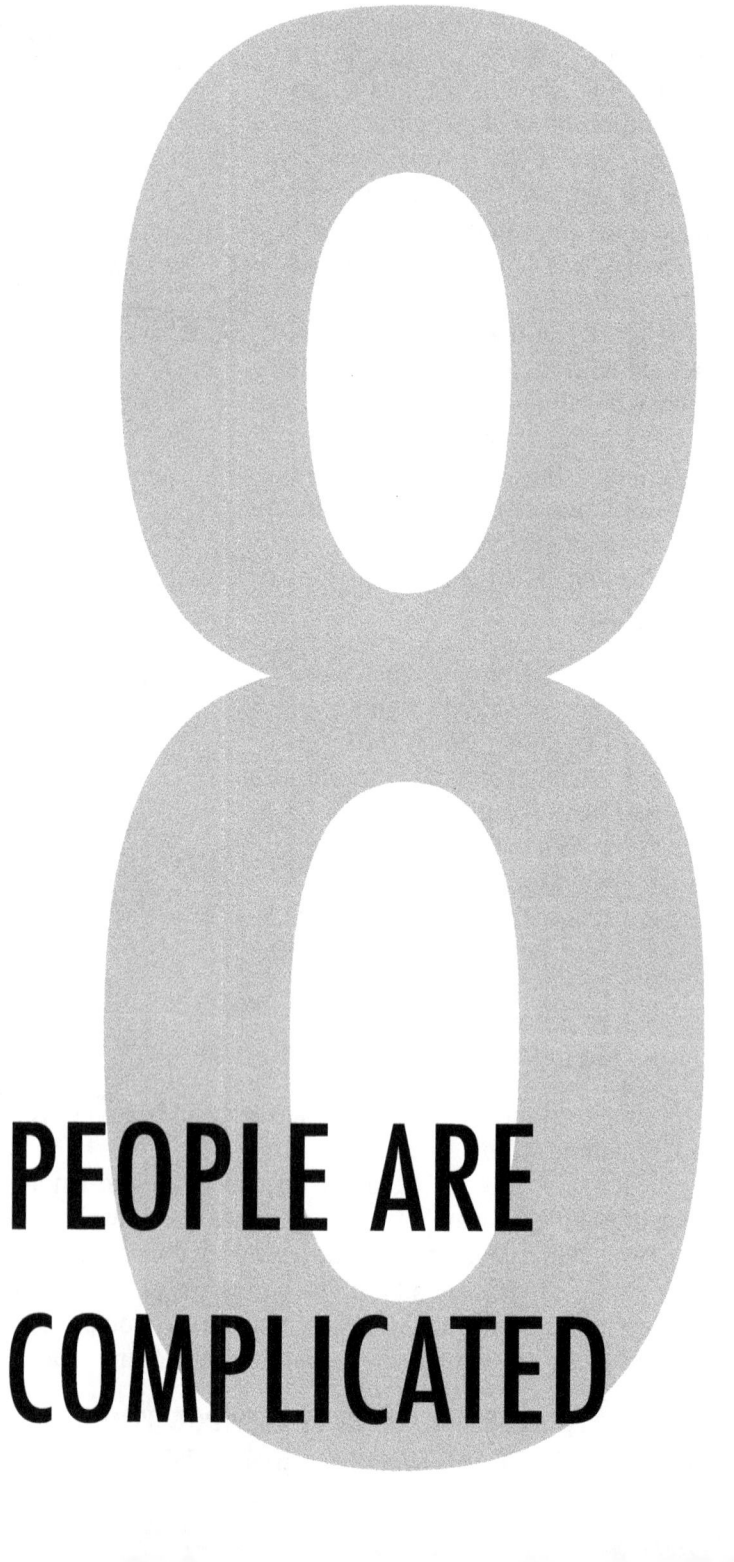

8
PEOPLE ARE COMPLICATED

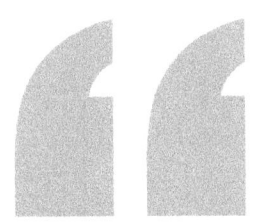

> You never really understand
> a person until you consider
> things from his point of view...
> until you climb inside of his
> skin and walk around in it.
>
> To Kill a Mockingbird - Harper Lee

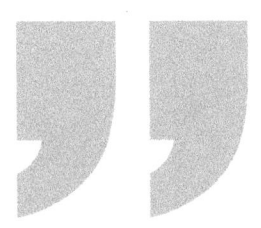

BOUNCER:
Be your own North Star,
the only one that matters.

Life is simple - People are complicated

How are you in physics? Compared to figuring out people, physics is a piece of cake. A teacher once told me that everything seems complicated until you understand it (profound eye roll). How easy is that... right? Does that imply that *eventually* you will understand everything... even physics? Um, no! Physics and I will never be close friends.

But life would be much easier if we could understand people and how they think. Psychologists have unsuccessfully tried to break the code for centuries. God purposely made each of us to be our own individual person. Even our voices are unique. But if we are all different, doesn't that complicate it more? Of course, but aren't you glad? Who wants to be a robot?

We will never completely understand people and how their minds work, even those we are the closest to... including ourselves. How well do you know you, or what you'll be thinking tomorrow? That's why I'm the worst packer ever when I travel. What if I packed red when I feel like black? Your mood can change, circumstances may change, or it could be those crazy hormones. You may hear someone say, "Oh, they would never do that. That's just not them," only to be utterly shocked when that person who would never do "that"... does it.

FIRST... NEVER "CULL" PEOPLE

My dad drilled oil wells out in the boondocks of Cornfield, USA. What he learned when working with investors was to never assume people couldn't afford to invest. "Don't ever cull people. You will miss a lot," he used to tell me. What he meant was to never count someone out based on your own assumptions.

One of my husband's favorite investors in commercial real estate is an older gentleman who drives a beat-up pick-up truck and wears worn flannel shirts and boots from another decade. When he sees a property he wants, he says, "Offer them $8 million and close in two weeks."

And he does. But if he asked you if he could borrow $100, based on his appearance, you would hesitate.

JUST WHEN YOU THINK YOU KNOW SOMEBODY

A great lady I worked with in my corporate life was the epitome of sweet mystery. Someone I adored. Over time, we became great friends, and I can't think of her to this day without smiling. She was soft-spoken, with a throaty, contagious laugh that pulled you in. Her hair was conservatively pulled up in a little knot that complimented her long pencil skirts, button-up shirt, and of course, the little ribbon necktie. She presented as a professional–the proverbial strait-laced librarian. Even her name was demure. Carol. Yeah, girl, that's you. And you know what's coming.

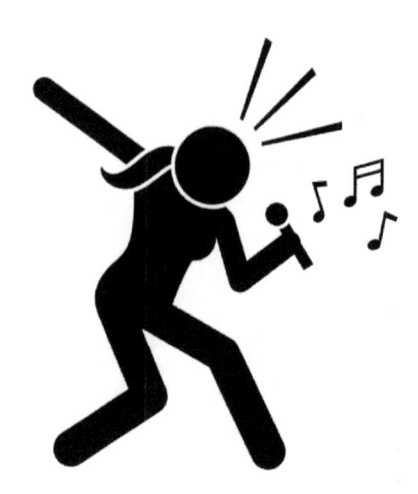

On a springy Saturday afternoon, we were having our annual corporate party on the huge blacktop parking lot outside our building. We had the customary parking lot food with adult beverages and a fabulous live band that featured amazing vocals accompanied by dynamic instrumentals, including horns. Nothing brings a party to life like a trumpet. The whole crowd was having a blast. While laughing with friends, I stopped dead in my tracks when I heard this fabulous gravelly voice belting out an incredible rendition of Mustang Sally. The female Wilson Pickett was right there in our parking lot. I looked at the others with big eyes that said, *"Where is this coming from?"* as I whipped my head around to see... Carol! Demure, quiet, *wouldn't say you know what if she had a mouthful,* Carol. She was on the stage with her long beautiful hair swinging through the air and over her face, blue-jeaned hips grinding, microphone in hand, winking at me with a gotcha smile. I smiled back with a thumbs-up. I learned a lesson that day. As much as I loved Carol... after that, I loved her and that hidden ornery streak even more. So, this is how it's going to be, girlfriend. Soon after that, we were wearing Billy Bob teeth as we drove down the streets, hanging out the windows, and bar-hopping–laughing hysterically and probably not nearly as funny as we thought we were. "Don't ever cull people. You will miss a lot." Indeed.

NO FORMULA

Life would be much easier if there was a convenient formula to help you understand people. A coy smile + a subtle head shake, and a, "Hello, how are you?" = who in the heck knows! You will never figure out what is going on inside the heads of people regardless of how long you try.

1. Jessica squinted at me because she didn't like what I said or what I was wearing.

2. Jonathan didn't say hello. I knew he didn't like me.

3. Laura didn't respond to my text message, again. That confirms it.

STOP wasting your time.
STOP trying to understand them.
STOP trying to be what you think they want you to be.

99.999999999999% OF THE TIME, YOU WILL BE WRONG.

1. Jessica squinted because she forgot her glasses and was trying to see something across the room.

2. Jonathan didn't say hello because he's thinking about the presentation he's giving in fifteen minutes. He actually didn't even see you.

3. Laura hates to text and rarely checks her messages or has been busy with her kids.

DO YOU SEE ANYTHING ABOUT YOU IN THERE?

There are endless reasons people act the way they do, say the things they do, and respond to situations the way they do. And they change when you stir in a little daily life... like a ticker tape. If you could devise a magic formula to easily understand people, it would make life easier, maybe a little stodgy, but you would be rich. Be warned, though, many have tried... like Sigmund Freud. Too many variables with moving parts causing constant change make it impossible to stereotype anyone, in spite of all the self-help books that try to do so.

Nagatha is relentless, constantly making you believe she has all the answers and treacherously letting you know that they all revolve around you. She is always looking for ways to egg on trouble by creating critical thoughts in your head, but she is not a psychologist. She certainly doesn't understand what's going on in the minds of all these complicated people any more than anyone else. But she is a whiz at making you believe she can. Isn't she? Didn't I tell you about Jessica? And Jonathan? And Laura?

I had the pleasure of seeing Zig Ziglar, one of my favorite authors and motivational speakers. He is a powerfully inspiring master at picking you up at the bottom when he starts and leaving you at the top when he finishes. His power remains intact even from the grave through his 31 books, affirmations, and videos. One of his most successful books is called *See You at the Top*. It is filled with humorous stories about biscuits, fleas, and pump handles, and that's where we are headed in Nagatha. You'll leave your critical inner voice at the bottom and arrive at the top without your uninvited roommate.

To quote Zig, getting your head on straight may require a Check-Up from the Neck-Up. Understanding people is the first step in winning the battle against Nagatha, starting with the most important person in your life. You. And it ain't easy! I can hear the groans now.

"Here we go. All about me and what I'm doing wrong. I'm the bad guy here. Right?"

Stay with me. It is essential that you learn to understand yourself, accept yourself, and like yourself... drum roll... JUST THE WAY YOU ARE! Minus the negative self-shaming thoughts. Hopefully, you will hear this mantra in your sleep.

"Yeah, yeah, yeah. Read that somewhere on a poster and I've already tried it. Doesn't work."

No one said it was going to be easy. You don't just wake up one day and say, "I'm going to start liking myself today." Do you even know what that means? If it was that easy, the whole world would be rainbows and lollipops.

"Yep, here I go... ready for your pep talk I've been meaning to give myself. You're a laugh a minute. Besides, I like me just the way I am."

No, you don't, or you wouldn't be here. Now STOP with the PLM pity party. If you want the easy way out, the just add water and the POOF approach that makes life magically peachy, you can throw this book over your shoulder and continue to live with Nagatha. *She's not so bad after a few years. You'll get used to the punches.*

Okay, let's hear it.

LET'S START IN THE KITCHEN

Think of it like making these great muffins you're going to love in the end... you must have flour, eggs, sugar, vanilla, and oil... or you just have an empty bowl. You get what you put into it. Listen and learn, practice and retrain your mind, throw out the old way of thinking and replace it with the right way. Welcome to Nagatha Boot Camp.

These are your ingredients:

- **Drill One:** Knowledge
- **Drill Two:** You can't change people. But you can change yourself, your perspective, and even your brain.
- **Drill Three:** Control your thoughts instead of allowing others to control them, and you control your life.

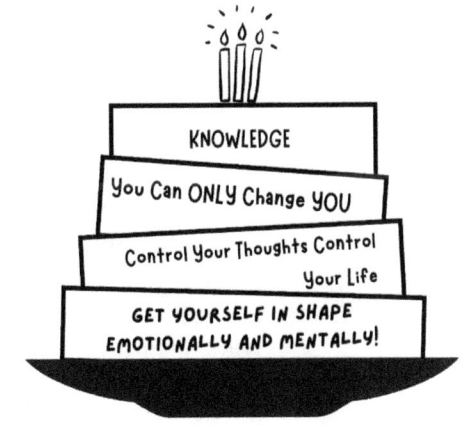

KNOWLEDGE

You Can ONLY Change YOU

Control Your Thoughts Control Your Life

GET YOURSELF IN SHAPE EMOTIONALLY AND MENTALLY!

- **Drill Four:** Get yourself in top shape emotionally and mentally, then kick out *Big Mouth–your adversary*.

People are complicated and you are one of them. If there was an easy way to understand them, it would be a pretty mundane world made up of *Stepford Wives*. They were somewhere between the Flintstones and Ed Sullivan. June Cleaver would come close?

For starters, there are the Type A personalities–the extroverted, high-energy people who are always on overdrive (that would be me). The more introverted laid-back ones are Type B. If stereotyping people into two categories was all there was to it, problem solved. She's a Type A, so I need to be bubbly and outgoing, maybe a touch of pushy, and ready to rock and roll for her to like me. But he's a Type B, so time to change my hat and be more quiet, careful not to alienate with intimidation.

Have you found yourself trying to get along with others by changing your persona to be like them? I certainly have. But what happens when you just want to be yourself? Do you want to change who you are to get along with people? What if they do the same? You are being the outgoing bubbly personality to get along with A and they are being what they think they need to be to get along with you, and... STOP this merry-go-round and let me off!

Now that we're off that merry-go-round, let's talk about what makes people so complicated. This will help you better understand WHY some people wouldn't like you.

KABOOM! Did you just say that? I don't need to hear it from you, I hear it day and night from Nagatha.

Exactly, but the truth is how you conquer giants. Did you think I was going to coddle you and tell you, "Oh, gee whiz, that's not true! Not only do they like you... but who couldn't love you, honey?" What's the point? More lies from me coupled with the lies you are hearing from Nagatha won't help you evict her and get to your destination–a place where you can peacefully live a long and happy life!

When you finish Nagatha Boot Camp, you will become your biggest fan, someone who can confidently tell themselves that not everybody likes them and feel happy about it.

"People are more complicated than the masks they wear in society."

—Robert Greene

YOU CAN'T PLEASE EVERYONE
YOU ARE NOT A MAGICIAN
YOU ARE HUMAN

And there lies your answer to why people are complicated. Looking too all-together, too composed, and overly confident is an offensive move. Intimidate or be intimidated. I've been there. The lady at the tea. Have you? Recognizing this in yourself is a big step in recognizing it in others and, consequently, understanding people. There's a good chance others haven't had the chance to find out if they like you... because they haven't seen the real you... and most likely, you aren't seeing the real them. Have the fortitude to unveil and be your wonderful self. Your new world of acceptance will disable your fear.

FLIP YOUR SELFIE ACTIONS:

1. Think about the part of you that you keep hidden from others... and why.

2. Have you been surprised by misreading someone you thought you knew? Describe the person you thought you knew and who you found out they were. Repeat as you think of others. What did you learn by doing this exercise?

3. Have you culled someone only to discover you were wrong about them? This is different from the second exercise. This is about judging someone by the way they look or act and making assumptions.

4. In what ways do you think people are complicated? Does that affect how you try to fit in and be liked?

9
SOME PEOPLE ARE JUST MEAN

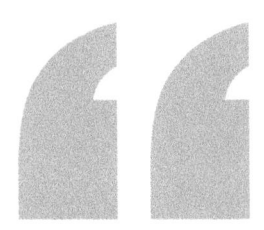

> The moment you feel you have to prove your worth to someone is the moment to absolutely and utterly walk away.

— Alysia Harris

BOUNCER:

It takes grace to remain kind when people are cruel.

PEOPLE CAN BE MEAN. DON'T TAKE IT PERSONALLY.

IT SAYS NOTHING ABOUT YOU BUT A LOT ABOUT THEM.

Sitting alone one evening, years ago, I lit some candles and dimmed the lights to enjoy the quiet as I looked out the window with a glass of wine, still numb from the events of a painful divorce from an abusive situation. At least I was beyond the years of torment and upheaval that occurred behind closed doors. The act was over. The future had to be brighter. The ringing of my phone broke the silence and jerked me back to reality. When I cautiously said hello, the husky disguised voice of a young woman asked, "Is it better by candlelight?" Then a few giggles in the background followed by a click.

Let the gossip begin... a new torment replacing the old. People can be mean.

If you're trying to convince yourself that all people are actually nice and have good intentions because... that's what the free spirits are spouting... get over it. I've witnessed some of the same "peace and love ya brother" free spirits throwing rocks when their cause was challenged, not caring if one landed on your deserving head. That's not to say there are not a lot of nice people in this world... because there are.

Do you ever get your fill of Kumbaya? Oh, go build a campfire!

- Everything is wonderful.
- Everyone is beautiful.
- Peace, not war.
- Happy! Happy! Happy!

STOP beating yourself up if you don't feel this way all the time, if you're angry, if you don't think everything is wonderful, and... you don't believe everyone is beautiful. You're not wrong. Put a sock in it,

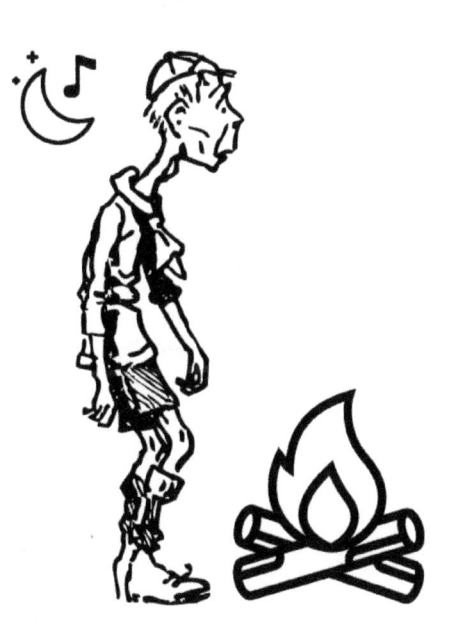

> "You do not wake up one morning a bad person. It happens by a thousand tiny surrenders of self-respect to self-interest."
>
> —Robert Brault

Ray! As much as I love your "beautiful" song and its uplifting message, it's a downer if you are dealing with "Nobody Likes Me Syndrome," feeling like a failure because everything is not beautiful in your life. For people who are hurting, putting on the mask of a beautiful song only hides the pain. It doesn't make it go away. All this happiness everywhere shoved down our throats can dump a guilt trip on us and make us feel we are a flawed outlier. Does that mean we should stop singing? Of course not. Let's not be cynical-just-throw-me-off-a-cliff. Just don't miss the line after everyone is beautiful... in their own way. Understand the reality that everything is not beautiful for anyone all the time. We all have our not-so-beautiful moments. This is real life, and you are normal. Normal.

WHY ARE PEOPLE MEAN?

Life is not wonderful for many people. It's hard. They may be dealing with sickness, poverty, anger from a history of abuse, depression, job loss... the list is endless. When I interviewed hundreds of people about their experiences growing up, it opened a door of understanding about why so many have the problems they do and why people can be mean. Very few felt they grew up in a happy, healthy environment.

Most grew up with abuse, anger, uninvited and unexpected hardships, and even mental illness. And yet they survived. Their shield of self-esteem intact but marred. Sanity safely holding fast deep inside. They overcame—just like their parents and generations before. Family dysfunction can be hereditary. But survival often meant their brain-created defense mechanisms. It also meant that some became warriors, learning to fight back. Learning to be tough. Deflecting their pain and uncertainties outwardly (to rebuild their self-respect and preserve their self-interest) sometimes manifests as mean.

We never know why everything is not beautiful for some people. We don't know what they are dealing with in their lives and why they seem complicated. People who abuse others, including their spouse, girlfriends, boyfriends, innocent children, co-workers, or others, are not beautiful. But neither are the ones who have abused them at some point in their lives to make them the way they are. They live on a battleship that's not easily turned. But what we do know is... it's not about us.

IT'S NOT ABOUT US

When you encounter someone who is mean, remind yourself that they are mean for a reason. Maybe they didn't have a role model to show them how to handle difficult, painful situations, or love them through it–a phrase I've shared countless times. Perhaps they need a shoulder, an ear, a little advice or understanding... or maybe just a hug that makes them feel they are special. Being made to feel worthy can even turn a battleship.

MEAN PEOPLE OR JUST HURTING

From the beginning of time, there have been mean, nasty people... for whatever reason. Every movie, even cartoons, has them. They could be mean for a myriad of reasons–the way they were raised, they had a mean parent as a role model, bad breaks in life, were beaten down mentally and physically by a caregiver, abused their whole life, or were continuously labeled growing up as a worthless, horrible, mean person. And because of it, they feel inferior around others. Mean can be a disguise hiding pain, embarrassment, or feelings of inadequacy. It's the defense mechanism that shields them.

But how many movies have the nasty mean character ending up being a good person in the end after something life-changing happens? Like when they are shown that someone cares about them or they inadvertently save the day and become the hero. Turns out they weren't mean

> "The person with the greatest hopes, the best outlook, has the greatest influence."
>
> —Christy Sawyer, <u>Arise and Shine My Love</u>

and nasty at all, just hurting and suffering on the inside from not having a caregiver or someone early in their life who built their self-esteem or self-confidence. Or perhaps they had a parent figure who, by example, wrongly taught them to act out their pain by hurting others... because they were hurting too and that's how they were taught.

IT'S NOT PERSONAL

It's not fun or easy for anyone to be around a mean person who is blatantly nasty and biting. When they direct their warfare at us, we naturally take their actions personally. But their mean isn't about you. You are just handy. Those who are dealing with NLMS are especially vulnerable.

Jerry Baily was a friend of mine in college... a great guy with an open heart. I was boo-hoo-ing to him one day, having a PLM pity party and sharing an upsetting something that someone had said to me. He just looked at me and smiled as he pulled a smooth, flat stone out of his pocket and placed it in my palm—a special gift—something he cherished. I'll never forget the look on his face. He wore the sweetest smile, one that crinkled his eyes and spread across his face. A smile that made everything okay. He said, "This is a worry stone, one I've had for a long time. Keep it close, and when you get upset, rub your thumb over it and say to yourself, 'No one is good enough to get me down." I've lost track of the countless times I've told myself that over the years and it always gets me through a tough time. Jerry, I

> "People don't dislike you for what you are. They don't like you for what they aren't."
>
> —Arvey Krise

want you to know how many lives you touched that day... I paid it forward. Thank you from us all. I hope you are doing great wherever you are today.

There will always be mean people who will try to use you to make themselves feel better. Don't let them. It's never about you. It's always about them. If you allow it, it won't help them feel better, instead, it will cause two people to feel bad about themselves. Try to understand their pain, knowing that *there for the grace of God go I*. It could be you. And remember, nobody is good enough to get you down.

FLIP YOUR SELFIE ACTIONS:

1. Has someone been mean to you in some way that affected the way you feel about yourself?

2. If someone is mean to you, do you see them as the one in the wrong? Or do you see yourself as deserving of what they've said or done? If not, how would you change it?

10 THE POWER OF YOUR CRITICAL INNER VOICE

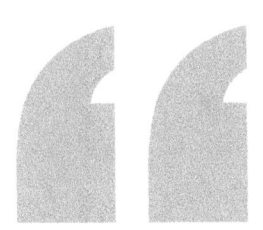

> The Biggest War of Life Resides Within Us...
>
> And it is only WE who can save US from OURSELVES!

- Lines of Insane Heart: By Madina

THE BATTLE WITHIN OURSELVES

It's time to get to work

This is where the rubber hits the road

This is where you put ON the gloves

This is where you get mentally and emotionally muscled up

THIS IS NAGATHA'S WATERLOO

THIS IS NAGATHA BOOT CAMP

I didn't know what it was. I just knew I had to have an answer. Then, one day, I started looking, asking questions, reading books, searching online about what I was doing wrong. Why didn't people like me? What I discovered was quite by accident. In that moment, I had hope... for the first time.

I *used to be* an inmate, locked up behind bars, a guest of the "Critical Inner Voice Prison." Alarmingly, it was located inside my own head. I felt there was no escaping this *life sentence*... until I found the key that unlocked the door to freedom. I walked through, leaving the warden, Nagatha, behind. All of us are fighting a never-ending internal war of good vs. evil to some degree. Even with things as simple as desperately wanting to devour that whole coconut cream pie, or the entire bag of Lay's Waverly potato chips I just ate because my elbow got stuck in repeat mode. We have a devil on one shoulder saying, "Go for it!" vs. an angel on the other screaming, *"Think about those scales in the morning!"*

WE ALL HAVE AN INTERNAL WAR –
GOOD VS. BAD

Our internal war has two sides, one squad fighting for you and the good person you want to be vs. the other squad fighting *against* you and the good person it doesn't want you to be. It's a battle you can win with the right strategy and information–like knowing your enemy, their game plan, and where they attack.

SQUAD A
THE GOOD GUY ON YOUR TEAM

Squad A is the positive side, which consists of your unique characteristics, positive traits, and emotional temperament. All the good things you inherited and have worked so hard to be. It wants only good things for you that will make you happy with high self-regard for who you are, and behavior you are proud of, like a friendly outgoing personality, a desire to be close in relationships, and a compassionate, loving view of yourself. Squad A is on your team, striving for you to be secure and confident, always fighting for you to accomplish your goals and have a healthy attitude toward the meaning of your life. Squad A is the nice guy. Its weapon is clear vision, knowledge, and the truth.

SQUAD B
NAGATHA — YOUR CRITICAL INNER VOICE

Nagatha is your antagonist, aka the villain. You are the protagonist... the hero of your own story. Except, this is real life, not fiction. I introduced you to her earlier and gave you the preliminaries like where she originated, BUT you don't know her... yet. This is where I take you behind the scenes and expose her covert operation with all the tendrils that can make your life miserable. What I discovered was frightening, and may be for you as well, especially when you realize that her base of operation is in your head. But knowing is enlightening, like a whoosh that suddenly opens your eyes... the wow moment when you step into a new world–your real world.

Nagatha is <u>*all things negative*</u> that you feel, the commander of Squad B, your internal enemy.

She's the mean-spirited fallen angel, the part of you that is fighting against you.

She's not to ever be confused with your conscience. It would never spur self-hatred.

She's the part of your personality that encourages and strongly influences self-destructive thoughts and behavior.

She's the little girl who nobody liked, who struck back... all grown up now.

Your *unleashed* critical inner voice is POWERFUL. A force to be reckoned with... AND so much more than the voice of NLMS. Nagatha is behind all things destructive or painful in your mind. The belittling, sneering, self-berating voices you hear are not hallucinations. They are indeed the voice of Nagatha... BUT they are only the tip of the iceberg, the visible little pieces of a much larger, deeply hidden enemy within each of us that causes the damage you never imagined your Nagatha was responsible for.

What's even more unnerving is how well your critical inner voice knows you, your unique personality, your unique weaknesses, and where to strike. It makes sense since it's been an integral part of you your whole life.

According to psychologists, Jay Earley and Bonnie Weiss, there are seven types of inner critics–the perfectionist, the taskmaster, the inner controller, the guilt tripper, the destroyer, the sabotager, and the molder. One of these is the most effective in damaging you.

YOUR NEW MANTRA—IT'S NOT ME

For much of my life, I was angry and didn't know why. I was full of all the self-everything negatives: self-blame, self-hate, self-destruction, self-failure, self-fault, and more, just putting self in front of all the bad feelings I cursed myself for. Looking back, I invented a lot of self-labels for things that weren't my fault. I didn't know why, but I knew that all of them came down to... yep... me. I was just not likable or wanted by anybody. But then something life-changing happened, as it will for you. I discovered the depth of the problems in my head that Nagatha is responsible for. They went above and beyond the disparaging thoughts we are aware of and then it all made sense. Like a scene in a movie when the protagonist finds the secret in the big hidden book in the basement, I whispered to myself, "Well, I'll be damned." My new bouncer became... it's not me.

EARTH-SHATTERING REVELATION... CRITICAL THOUGHTS ARE JUST THE BEGINNING OF THE HAVOC CAUSED BY NAGATHA

How many times do we have a toothache only to find out we need a root canal? Sometimes what's on the surface can be indicative of much bigger problems lurking below that can be a game-changer. Like now. From my own experience, I can tell you the self-punishing lies of your critical inner voice are just the tip of the problems it's causing–there are also ones you didn't even know were related. Using your new mantra, It's Not Me, you can fight Nagatha and win when you experience:

- Times when you suddenly feel sad, anxious, or in a bad mood and it causes a negative shift in your emotions without you understanding why

- Unsettling thoughts advocating negative actions contrary to your well-being

- Personalizing things by making them your fault, causing you to feel worthless and not good enough

- Self-punishing thoughts and an attitude that diminishes your self-esteem

- Hostility towards not only yourself but others

- Believing negative thoughts that lead to maladaptive behavior

- Magnifying potentially negative situations and feeling worse than you should

- Varying degrees of unfounded anger and sadness

- Self-limiting behavior that prevents you from reaching goals and sabotages your best interests

- Polarizing thoughts that ignore positives and focus on negatives (like thinking someone hates you when they don't call you back)

- Hostile, cynical attitudes that tend to warn you about other people
- A negative, pessimistic picture of the world
- Undermining your ability to interpret events realistically
- Feeling distant and alienated that sometimes leads to isolation

THE FIRST STEP IN WINNING IS TO STOP AND LISTEN!

FRIENDLY CHATTER IS NECESSARY

We all hear 'head chatter' that talks to us on an ongoing basis. Good voices in our head are normal, and according to mental health experts, keep us sane. They keep us company when we are alone, like walking on a treadmill or working on a project. They help us think through scenarios and make decisions about... well, everything. What to wear, the red dress or the comfortable jeans. What to cook for dinner, the pot roast or the pancakes. Sometimes the voices just pop out of our mouths and we find we are talking out loud to ourselves. When I accuse my husband of not listening to me, he says, "Well, how am I supposed to know you're talking to me? You're always talking to yourself!" Really? Your task is to know the difference between the good (your friends and comrades you need and want to keep close by), and the bad that beats us up and even leads us to withdraw socially. It's easy to differentiate, but it takes being on the lookout and nailing them.

I FELT HELPLESS... UNTIL I DISCOVERED THE POWER OF ME

WINNING AGAINST NAGATHA

There are three typical responses to Nagatha:

> "I have self-doubt. I have insecurity. I have fear of failure. I have nights where I show up at the arena and I'm like, 'My back hurts, my feet hurt, my knees hurt. I just want to chill.' We all have self-doubts."
>
> —Kobe Bryant

1. You are not even aware of it, which means it's controlling your mind without you realizing it.

2. You believe and agree with what it's saying and follow its dictates.

3. You argue with it ineffectively as it strengthens its power over you.

WINNING THE BATTLE

- CHALLENGE NAGATHA when she fills your mind with critical admonitions. By telling yourself it's not true and believing it, you empower yourself to take control, consciously shutting her down with your new weapon–knowledge.

- Take away the power of her destructive thoughts by 1) identifying them, and 2) becoming acutely aware of what they are telling you. Only then can you break away from your usual behavior and choose how you respond.

- STAY OUT OF THE PAST. IT'S GONE.

- Calm your mind and BE in the here and now. Being present in this way is called mindfulness. Your critical inner voice (Nagatha) is from your past and has no business being in the present.

- LET GO RATHER THAN GIVING CRITICAL COMMENTS AN EAR.

- Don't gift any of your valuable time to self-destructive thoughts. Instead, dismiss them with arrogance and send them back to where they came from.

- Out-persist them with self-lifting thoughts. Call in your bouncers and bounce them out.
- STAND YOUR GROUND WITH CONFIDENCE.
- STOP ARGUING... I learned a long time ago that you can't argue with a drunk. Words to live by.
- Hold to your beliefs: I like me. I love me. Believe in who you are and hold tightly to those convictions.
- Walk away.
- Sometimes you have to stop wasting your energy and agree to disagree!

THE TWO WOLVES

A Cherokee elder was teaching his young grandson about life.

"A fight is going on inside me," he said to the boy. "It is a terrible fight, and it is between two wolves. One is evil. He is anger, envy, sorrow, regret, greed, arrogance, self-pity, guilt, resentment, inferiority, lies, false pride, superiority, self-doubt, and ego.

The other is good. He is joy, peace, love, hope, serenity, humility, kindness, benevolence, empathy, generosity, truth, compassion, and faith.

This same fight is going on inside you—and inside others, too."

The boy thought about it for a minute and then asked his grandfather,

"Which wolf will win?"

The elder simply replied, "The one you feed."

(A legend of unknown origin.)

FLIP YOUR SELFIE ACTIONS:

Experts say that of the 25,000-60,000 thoughts we have a day, 90 percent of them are negative.

1. Get paper and pen and write down all Nagatha's critical, painful thoughts. I.e., I'll never get that job. I don't belong. Nobody likes me.

2. Make a check mark by the ones that have led you to destructive behavior or detoured you from a goal. Take a few minutes and study the list, especially the ones with a check beside them.

3. Now wad up the paper and destroy it along with those thoughts. They're gone.

4. Which wolf are you feeding?

PART III

ABOUT DISCERNING YOU: THE GOOD GUY

11
IT'S ALWAYS BEEN YOU

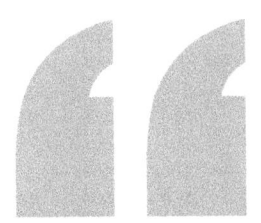

> The truth is scary, but knowing
> nothing is crippling.
>
> - Becca Fitzpatrick

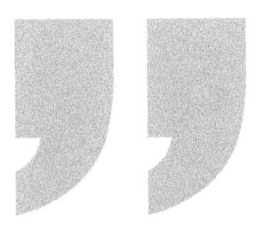

BOUNCER:
I'm the director and producer of my own show.

I love horror movies, which is probably the reason I'm terrified to stay alone at night. Stephen King is the king of fright. REDRUM REDRUM. I thought I was going to wet my pants watching *The Shining*... all six times. But one of the scariest movies I remember from years ago is *Sorry, Wrong Number*. A young woman home alone on a dark, stormy night (of course) is getting phone calls from a man whispering terrifying threats.

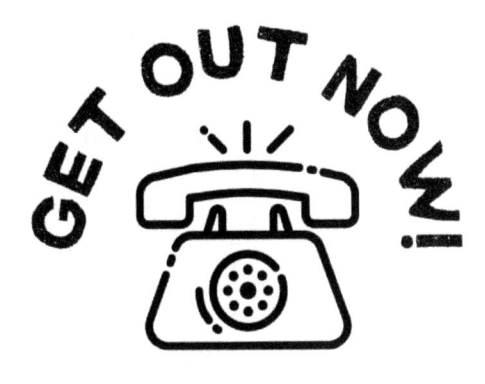

"I'm watching you."

She frantically calls the police. A few minutes later, they call her back screaming,

"The call is coming from inside your house. Get out now!"

THE BIG REVEAL

This chapter is the twist in your horror movie.

It's the moment you discover the blood-sucking tick that has been quietly nestled in your hair, getting fatter and more content while you've felt worse and worse.

It's the Big Reveal of the monster that has been living in your house... that you didn't know was there.

It's the moment you understand and win.

It's what this book is about, understanding why we feel that nobody likes us and why we anguish over it, allowing it to control our thoughts, our joy, our peace of mind, our behavior, and... our lives.

It's about making it go away.

And just like my little six-year-old in the chapter, Why Do I Need to be Liked?, it's about a life-changing new perspective called... reality.

A philosophy class called critical thinking was one of my college favorites. We were given brain teasers to solve. To find the answer, you had to get lost in your thinking, just you and the riddle, seeing possible solutions scribbled on an imaginary wall in your head as confusion loomed, enveloping you while your brain came up with one scenario after another. Then a light bulb came on and the answer materialized in a surreal moment like it had been there all the time. Then the hard part... translating it to others so they could fully understand.

After years of trying to understand why nobody liked me, the light bulb came on in the middle of the night. I wanted to run up and down the street in my nightgown, screaming from the newfound freedom I felt. Like a not-guilty verdict after a grueling trial. Something I had stashed away years ago when studying psychology surfaced, and it all made sense. I was deliriously happy, full of a sense of knowing. And so much peace. Beautiful, soothing, inner peace. After years of research and studying, I had found it... the missing piece of the puzzle. I had finally discovered the treasure map that put me on the right road to my destination, evicting Nagatha. Now to explain it.

THE MISSING PIECE – PEACE

You have been looking in the wrong place. It's not that nobody likes you. Outside of the norm (yes, you are the norm), these self-massacring feelings have nothing to do with other people. Chances are they like you just fine, and that's if they have even thought about it or know you. Like the name of the movie, you have a wrong number.

You are projecting. It's a defense mechanism people use when they unconsciously take *unwanted emotions* or *traits they don't like about themselves* and attribute them to someone else. A married woman who can't admit her feelings of being attracted to another man jealously accuses her husband of flirting and being attracted to other women. A parent who thinks of themselves as a failure tells their child they will never amount to anything. A man who feels insecure about his masculinity mocks other men who have effeminate behaviors. A person who doesn't like themselves accuses others of not liking them.

The reason you look at others and convince yourself that they don't like you, even falsely interpreting their actions as proof, is that you don't like yourself... you attribute an unwanted emotion within yourself to others.

THE CALL IS COMING FROM INSIDE THE HOUSE. YOUR HOUSE.

Discovering that the monster behind my agony was living inside my head was a shocking but welcome revelation, as it should be for you, too. Because now that you know, you can take control and fix it. You can't leave the house like the girl in the movie, but you can kick the caller out of the house by taking back the reins from Nagatha, the one who is pulling the strings of the monster. How do you do that? When you learn to like yourself, Nagatha will move out.

NOW YOU KNOW.
IT'S ALWAYS BEEN YOU.

12
YOUR POWERFUL CIRCLE

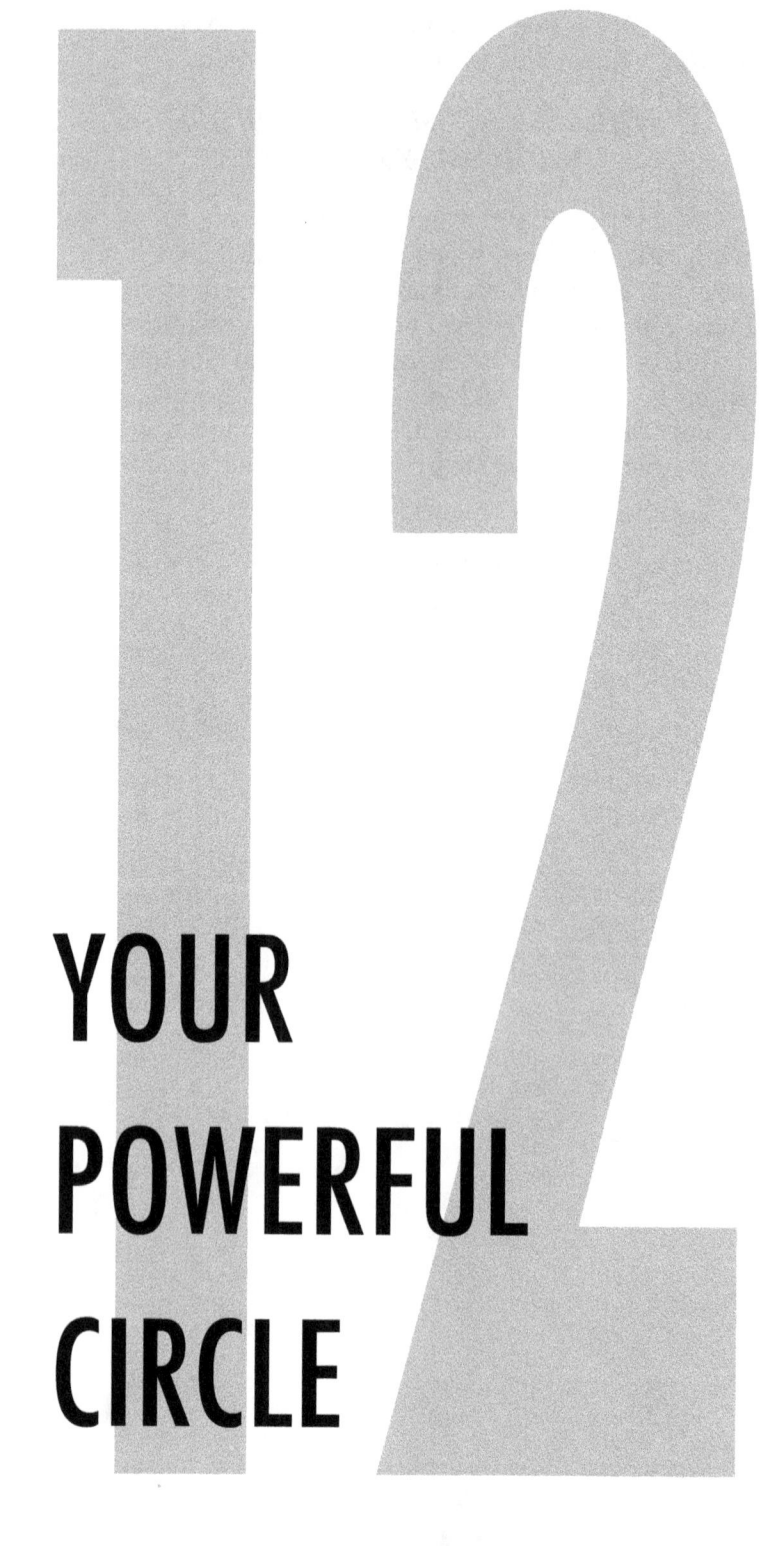

> The greatest reflection of priorities is your time. Whatever you say about what matters to you, the true test is where you place your time.
>
> - Nick Crocker

BOUNCER:
You don't freely give time or space... you are robbing it from someplace else.

Think of a good cup of coffee. Can you smell the aroma? Rich and full of flavor. It's that *Ahhhh* moment. Puts you into a really happy place, doesn't it? Maybe grab a good book, or newspaper, watch your favorite show. Heaven.

But it was so good that, next time, you grabbed a bigger cup, a huge cup, and you added extra water to the brew. You wanted more. Make it last longer... go further. After all, isn't more better?

But there's a problem. A serious problem. The coffee grounds were stretched too far, expended, and that rich, bold cup of coffee is gone. So diluted that it lost its bold, rich flavor. It's no longer a good, inviting cup of coffee you can enjoy, one that makes you feel wonderful and curls your toes as you spend time reading that book or newspaper. All of that extra water took away the meaning of a good cup of coffee. It lost its taste, the Ahhh moment. It's no longer valuable or even something you want.

Is this you? Always adding more water to your already perfect cup by wanting and needing more validation, obsessed with trying to be liked by *everyone*? Are you trying to add more rings to your powerful circle? As your time and energy become diluted, there's little left for the most important people in your life–you, your spouse, your children, your best friends, etc. Instead of focusing your time and energy on them, you reach out to everybody, people you don't even know who mean nothing to you, consumed with trying to please them, be liked by them, and be everything to everyone. You go places you don't want to go, join organizations you don't want to join, and soon, you have nothing left to give. You are used up, out of time and energy, and overwhelmed with your unwanted commitments.

You've spread yourself so thinly in your need to be liked by everyone that you have become that diluted cup of coffee. You've lost your flavor. You are no longer rich and robust for those in your powerful circle... or anyone else, including you.

Here's the real wake-up call! It may surprise and even disappoint you but... drum roll... you are not superhuman. Yeah, I'm talking to you. It's reality, a revelation you are going to have to live with. You are just a common mortal like the rest of us... not Mork–for those of you who remember the hilarious alien on *Mork and Mindy*. Shouting "Nanu, Nanu!" and even doing the Vulcan handshake can't rustle up a few more hours of boundless energy in a day, any more than twitching your nose can. How many worried mothers called their family pediatrician concerned that their daughter had a neurological condition that caused her to repeatedly twitch her nose and squint her eyes, only to be told she was a wannabe witch like Samantha on the hit sitcom, *Bewitched*? After hours of practice in my grandma's little den on Thursday nights, not a single frog to show for it! Luckily for my tormenting little brother.

YOU ARE THE RINGMASTER

WHAT'S IN YOUR POWERFUL CIRCLE (YPC)?

Think of your life as a finite circle that represents all your time and energy. It has a border, a *boundary* that says enough, that's all there is, and protects you from spreading yourself too thinly. As hard as you may try, it doesn't stretch or move. It's a *boundary*.

Imagine this circle as a target with a big round red circle in the middle that is you. You are the center because it's your circle, your life, so everything in it revolves around you. Around you are rings that represent where you allot your time and energy. The first ring is closest to you and represents your first priority for where you allot your time and energy. Around it is a second ring, followed by a third ring, and it continues until the circle is full. Each ring that is added moves further away from you as they go further down the list of your priorities. The depth of each ring will depend on how full it is of people and commitments, and how demanding they are of your time. You may only have one person in any given ring, like your spouse, for instance, who requires more of your time than another with a hundred, each requiring little. Your Powerful Circle

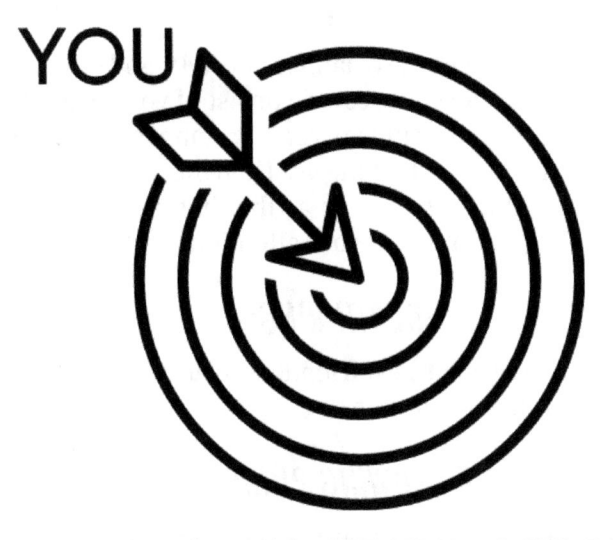

YOUR POWERFUL CIRCLE

clearly defines and gives order to your priorities—and you are the ringmaster.

Everyone's Powerful Circle is their own—unique to them and their life. They are the CEO and determine who they allow in and where they are placed in their circle.

This is an example of how yours may look:

CENTER:

Circle, which is you, the bullseye.

FIRST RING:

Those closest to you, likely your spouse or significant other.

SECOND RING:

If you are a parent, this one probably contains your children.

(Most people will spend most of their time and energy in the first two rings. You might choose to merge them into one—it's your ring.)

THIRD RING:

Depending on family dynamics, lifestyle, and other circumstances, the next ring could consist of your extended family, which might include parents, grandparents, brothers, sisters, nieces, and nephews. Thought: They may not be as demanding of your time as the first two: Extended family can require much of your attention.

FOURTH RING:

This could be your best friend(s), relationships can be time-consuming to maintain.

FOLLOWING RINGS:

- After best friends, you may need to allot a ring for casual friends, one which may be very full and diversified.

- You'll most likely need a ring for work and job relationships. We all know how demanding these can be on your time and energy.

- Somewhere in your circle, there may be a ring for church and church friends, and perhaps one for relationships through kids' activities like dance or soccer.

- Then there is a bulging ring for acquaintances or other interests. You could label this catchall ring miscellaneous.

ARE YOU ASKING WHAT'S LEFT FOR ME?

That depends. There's another ring that can be a thief in the night, an intruder, robbing you of time and energy... an *everybody has to like me* ring. It could be at the beginning, middle, or end... depending on where it falls in your *list of priorities* and... how much time you spend there doing things just to make people like you. It's a short-lived ring. It will disappear after you evict Nagatha along with your needy needs.

This is a *self-determined* diagram of where you allocate your time and energy based on the priorities in your life during any given season. Created and fueled by your personal choices, it is subject to change as those priorities shift. Years ago, when Nagatha had me in her clutches with the NLMS, my priorities were different than they are today. I found myself rationalizing my choices, not recognizing them for what they were... a desperation to have more. I illogically believed that more would help me be included and accepted. I was blind to what was right in front of me, the happiness and fulfillment I already had. My hungry insecurities had to be fed.

I used to say that my life didn't stop because I had kids–guilt talking from a mother whose circle was too full. When I flipped my selfie and realized that my meaningful life only started when I had kids, I took inventory and "cleaned the circle." That's when my rings shifted. The rings in YPC and their members will change throughout your life as you pass through your seasons–kids grow up, jobs change, demands on your time shift. Only you can man the controls. You are the gatekeeper; you decide who you let into your circle at any given time. Life is not stagnant. Your circle has a pulse until you die, but these **power words** *will always be significant in your life*

UNDERSTAND THE "DYNAMISM" OF POWER WORDS IN YPC

Choose = Control

Choice = Freedom

Integrity = Self-esteem

Allow others to choose = Forfeit control

Trade-offs = Cost or gain

Decision = Power

Courage = Live Your Life Your Way

Values = Your Values, Your North Star

No talk = Listen

Boundaries = Protection

MAYBE I JUST NEED TO GET OUT MORE

Do you find yourself going through slumps, having *Nobody Likes Me* self-pity parties, feeling alone and sure that you don't have any real friends? We've all been there. I used to convince myself that the remedy was to get out and become more involved in the community. That had to be the problem. I had become too isolated from the real world. From people. Blame shift!

I tend to live in *full-steam-ahead gear. Did I mention not thinking it through* and immediately jumping in with the notorious *all fours*? Getting out meant not just joining one, but every organization that people I knew were in. The thing that makes it worse is... I hate meetings. I mean, I seriously detest them. Too many years in the corporate world being stuck on every committee because... you know... they had to have me because... hmmm. Schmooze, Schmooze. I knew I was going to hate *having* to go to all those meetings, but... it was a necessary evil if I was going to be liked by everybody.

But it gets worse! (How... you might be asking yourself?) The insane irrational thinking continues. Not being able to say *NO* for fear of *not being liked*, I found myself on committees. Committees I didn't want to be on, becoming officers of clubs I didn't want to belong to, and soon, not having time for the most important people in my Power Circle, including the one with the bobbing-bubble "Yes-Head"... ME!

Soon, memories of why I had previously fled these clubs came roaring back. Contrary to the persuasive bogus babble, I wasn't being asked to be on those committees or to be officers of those clubs because I was the best one to do the job. NOBODY ELSE WANTED TO DO IT!

OPPORTUNITIES CAN BE CODE FOR DEMANDS ON YOUR TIME AND ENERGY

Walking into a meeting of an industry organization for women, wearing my business suit and all of my teeth and fairly good grammar intact, I was given a target for my backside as I signed in. Soon enough, the build-you-up arrows were fired and hit me square dead center between my shoulders. Thank God I was there, an opportunity—sent from heaven above—to be their next president-elect. Perfect to lead this organization to the top with all of my experience and leadership skills. There was NO ONE else who had my credentials. I was their savior. I said NO. Thanks, but NO THANKS. I simply did not work in a volunteer leadership role with organizations... ESPECIALLY groups of women (sorry, but reality is a bummer) who, without fail, engage in fighting, back-stabbing, setting up camps, and callously gossiping with the intention of ruining each other. NO, THANKS. Oh... but we are different, they begged. No, you are not, I countered. After multiple coercion-blowing smoke-enticed breakfast meetings, I finally told them with a smirk that I would become their president-elect... however, at the first sign of "the above", I would be gone. And by the way, girls, you might want to hold off a bit on ordering my new name badge. I was 100 percent positive this would never come to fruition based on my non-negotiable conditions. I wasn't even sworn in before the trouble began. Although I felt bad for the incoming president who was the brunt of the unfair, selfishly motivated, heartless, cruel attacks by the low self-esteem, needy, out-going president, it wasn't my problem, and I had no intention of making it mine. With a smile, I excused myself from the office of president-elect and laughed all the way to my car. Lesson learned, girls. Being older with notches on my belt has its advantages. I had allowed them to slip into my Powerful Circle, into my everybody has to like me ring. As I realigned my priorities and closed the gate, I could hear their favorite word... NEXT!

When all my family and close relationships started to suffer because of me over-committing myself... I suffered the most... out of guilt for trying to nurse my self-pity wounds at their expense, and for making them feel less important. I beat myself up for missing things that meant the most to me and my loved ones, events that were happening in my powerful circle while I was busy for the wrong reasons. Misplaced priorities that led to wrong choices, resulted in sacrificed memories that could never be replaced. And for what? I got out of those commitments and went home. Home to my Powerful Circle...

- Powerful in my life and the lives of those in it.
- Powerful to my happiness and those I care about.
- Powerful to REAL and all that matters.

This is a humorous account of an actual event, not a hit on clubs and organizations. It's healthy, mentally and emotionally, to be involved with groups you enjoy... as long as you are not making trade-offs of time and energy you'll later regret. Give yourself permission to step away if need be and come back at a better time. Regret is a terrible feeling that hurts from head to toe. Be as kind and considerate to yourself as you would be to anyone else.

WOULD YOU INVEST YOUR MONEY WITHOUT KNOWING YOUR ROI?

If all you had to invest was $10,000 to determine the quality of your future, how would you invest it? Would you try to invest in everything, afraid you would miss an opportunity? Or would you choose to put your money where it would give you the greatest return on investment (ROI)? We plan for our future finances and retirement, but do we plan for our future relationships? Are you investing in the memories of your family? Kids don't forget. Have you ever thought about the *return on investment* of the time you spend with the important people in your life; about what both you and they are going to get out of it when it matures in the future? What do you want it to be? You probably have a pretty good idea of what your financial portfolio will look like when you retire, yet getting so wrapped up in your everyday NOW, it's easy to assume that nothing will ever change... until it's gone. Guilty as charged.

- I can work this in.
- There's plenty of time.
- Things will always be like they are today.
- My family will always be waiting for me when I'm finished with these commitments, the ones I've allowed into my Powerful Circle.
- I'll make it up to them and we'll do something special together... as soon as.

AS SOON AS - AS SOON AS - AS SOON AS - AS SOON AS - AS SOON AS

MY MOTHER WAS RIGHT — YOU BLINK AND IT'S GONE

I know, I know, I know. You've heard it all before. But do you believe it? Seems like you were chasing those busy toddlers forever until... you blinked, and they were gone. And you can never get that time back again. Don't wait for birthdays, graduations, and losses to open your eyes and, suddenly, you notice your little guy is a foot taller and heading into middle school... or college. The window of opportunity for your personal dreams has closed. You hear your mother say, "Where does the time go?" and you get a lump in your throat as you wipe away a tear and consider your ROI on how you spent that time... now gone. Was it a good investment? As much as you try to fulfill your needs, Nagatha will never be satisfied for as long as she lives upstairs in your mind. And she loves the new ammunition you've given her... guilt.

YOU ARE RICH

You may not know it, but... *you are rich!* Before you wonder, *"What did I miss?"* and check your bank account, please understand being rich isn't about money. It's about what's all around you. You've been an investor for a long time of the most important resource you have... your time. Will you invest it in building worthless short-term relationships? Or those that will be there for all your tomorrows? Misplaced priorities can blind you to the painful consequences of desperate choices. Lost time that can never be recovered.

As of right this moment, you have the awesome responsibility of choosing whether to make good... or bad... investments. Your future depends on the choices you make, starting today. Past doesn't matter. Your ROI can be a happy and healthy life if you invest wisely and build a strong portfolio full of great decisions.

ENOUGH IS ENOUGH...
STOP AND BE HAPPY

WHAT IF...

- We stopped competing with people we don't care about and quit buying more things we don't need with money we don't have to impress people we don't like?

- We STOP trying to impress people with how busy and important we are?

- We gifted ourselves the freedom of living life to make us happy vs impressing others, buying a house WE like because we want to, or selling a house and hitting the road because we want to?

I knew a couple who said what if... and did it. They sold their beautiful house, gave their furniture to their kids, and bought an Airstream to live and travel in. They gave themselves freedom, freeing themselves of burdensome responsibilities and putting their happiness first. Happy trails.

**UNDISCIPLINED PURSUIT OF MORE =
FAILURE**

SOME THINGS HAVE GOTTA GO!

THE POWER OF DECISIONS

How you manage YPC determines the richness of your life. The further you are stretched, the more diluted your time and energy becomes, and the less effective you will be. You can only be spread so far and still maintain the quality of your relationships.

Ask yourself:

- Do I have time to talk to my kids about their day over an ice cream cone after school?

- Can I give my husband my full attention when he's telling me about a problem?

- If your good friend is having a crisis, do you have time to sit with them and give them the uninterrupted ear they need?

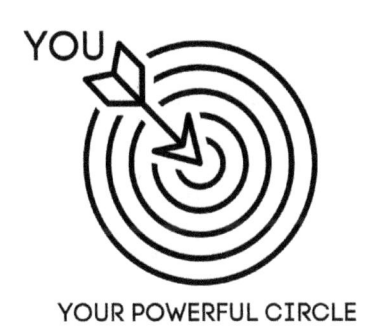

YOUR POWERFUL CIRCLE

Prioritizing means deciding what matters. Like the robust cup of coffee, full of rich and bold flavor, quality is much better than quantity. Only you have the power to allow others in or... kick them out. Give yourself the *freedom* and courage to unlock the door to *choose*. Decisions are work and require discipline. I'm the worst! "Are you ready to order?" Those five words throw me into a panic. When eating out with friends, it's a standing joke... take her order last *(I'll have page two please! So much easier than those dastardly decisions)*. And curse whoever invented chocolate ice cream when I was just fine with only vanilla!

Which of my creative ideas to include when writing keeps me awake at night. Luckily, my friend, Jon Acuff, off-the-chart speaker and very successful author of eight books and working, told me to think "next book". Stay tuned for my 49 books coming soon! Having a grip on your priorities will shield you from the unwanted consequences of rationalizing guilt-ridden choices.

> *I have lots of time.*
> *I'll make it up to them.*
> *They won't miss me, they're busy anyway.*

When faced with saying YES OR NO to another commitment, challenge your "I have to... can't say no" mentality and ask yourself:

- What's the cost?
- Who will I hurt?
- Is it important to me?
- If I had to do it today, would I do it? (If you don't want to do it today, you still won't want to do it tomorrow.)
- Who or what am I robbing time from?
- Will it overcrowd my Powerful Circle?

I've learned to listen to my gut. Having reservations means NO. Most commitments are trivial–few are vital.

WHAT OTHERS EXPECT DOESN'T MATTER IN THE END GAME.

BE TRUE TO YOURSELF AND YOUR VALUES.

LESS IS BETTER.

You can't squeeze in everyone without trade-offs. Who are you going to sacrifice? Your family, friends, or work? Know going in where you want to invest your time and energy. Like a diet, you can't wait until you are hungry to decide. Think of Your Powerful Circle like a cookie jar. When it's full, it's full. There *ain't no more room*. You can try to cram in more–but you'll end up with crumbs.

NO ROOM FOR BAD GUYS

Do you have anyone who has found their way into your circle that is sucking all the air out of the room–draining your energy dry? Beware of people who are robbing you of joy with their own negativism or demands and taking up valuable space. Occasionally, you need to do inventory and *Clean the Circle* (just like you clean your house), and rid YPC of the bad to make room for the good.

To quote Christie Sawyer in her book, *Arise, My Love*, what if you said, "Bitterness, you have to go because you're taking up space where peace could be," or if you looked at your misery and said, "You have to go because you're taking up space where my purpose could be," or looked at your depression and said, "You have to go because you're taking up space where my joy should be."

You must have the insight and *courage* to remove people (and/or commitments) from Your Powerful Circle that are impacting relationships and moments you can never replace. Is it time to clean out your cookie jar and throw away the crumbs?

PRACTICE ASKING YOURSELF,

"STAY OR GO?"

"YES OR NO?"

"LOTS OF GOOD THINGS OR A FEW GREAT THINGS?"

IF WE DON'T MANAGE OUR TIME AND ENERGY WITH PURPOSE, OTHERS ARE HAPPY TO MANAGE THEM FOR US.

YOUR CHOICE = YOUR PRIORITIES

OTHERS' CHOICE = THEIR PRIORITIES

Purposely choose where to focus... or forfeit the right and live with the consequences of someone else doing it for us.

Save time to enjoy the rich and bold flavors of what you have. Your happiness is right there inside of you. Everything else is just coffee grounds.

ON YOUR FINAL DAY, WHAT WILL YOU WISH YOU HAD DONE TODAY?

FLIP YOUR SELFIE ACTIONS:

1. Draw or copy your own empty diagram of Your Powerful Circle with you being the center, or copy the one in this book and enlarge it. You can add as many rings as you need to accommodate your lifestyle. Prioritize the rings around the center (you) with the people in the first one being those you are the closest to and spend most of your time with (i.e., your spouse), followed by the ones next on your list of priorities. This will take some time and serious thought to complete, but you will find it is a valuable tool. It can change your life by enabling you to evaluate where you spend your time and energy and help you determine if you have your priorities where you want them to be.

2. Keep a log for a month of where you spend your time, including who you are with (person, work,

or organization) and your purpose. At the end of the designated period, tabulate by categories and percentages, then compare that to the YPC you created.

3. Are they in sync? What changes do you need to make?
4. What's your ROI for where you delegate your time and energy?
5. What do you plan to do with your life?
6. When will you begin?
7. What are the bare bones of happiness and contentment for you and those you love?

YOUR POWERFUL CIRCLE

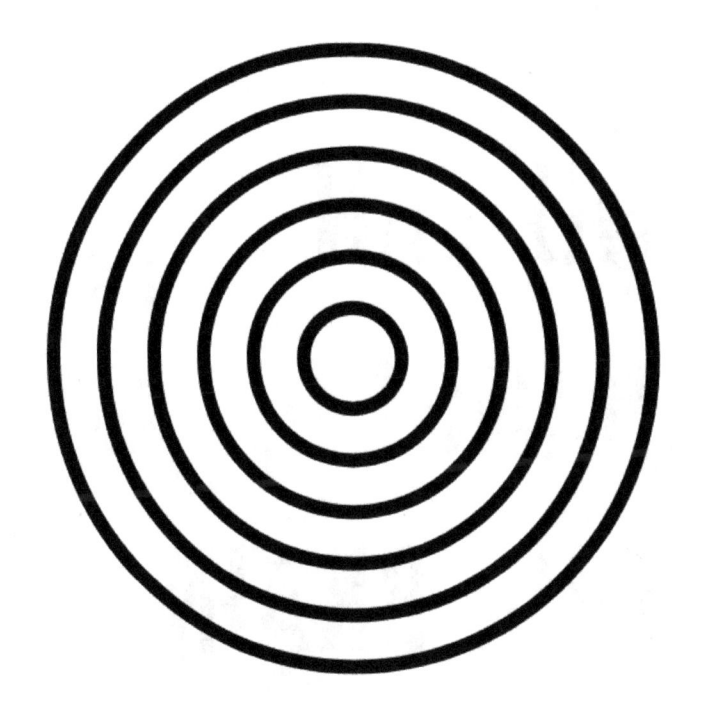

13
YOU CAN CHANGE YOUR BRAIN

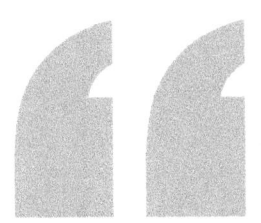

> The mind is the most restless,
> unruly part of mankind.
>
> - Sarah Young
> *Jesus Calling: Enjoying Peace in His Presence*

BOUNCER:
My brain is a personal computer I can reprogram.

CHANGE YOUR BRAIN?

Your brain is an amazing organ, the most intricate, complicated, and "mind-boggling" *computer* known to man. Scientists have tried to understand it and replicate it for years. But it seems that God is the all-time geek of geeks, the master in creating the human brain.

You may not be aware that your brain has a handy built-in option. It allows you to reprogram it if you don't like the way your OS is functioning. Like any computer whiz, you just have to know how... which buttons to push, which tabs to open and close, how to download the software you want to install, and how to delete the software you don't like.

The types of thoughts we think largely determine our state of mind. Makes sense... garbage in, garbage out as the saying goes, which is where your coach comes in. The conversations we have within ourselves are orchestrated by our own personal mind coach that directs our feelings and behavior. The problem starts when Nagatha moves in. When this happens, our limbic system (the *emotional brain*) becomes overactive, sending her critical thoughts down the *negative funnel*, straight to depression and despair. We then see things through a dark filter, resulting in feelings of regrets from our past and pessimism and anxiety about our future.

Psychiatrist Dr. Daniel G. Amen, MD, founder of the world-renowned Amen Clinics and author of more than ten New York Times best sellers, refers to these cynical, gloomy, and complaining thoughts that just keep coming by themselves as ANTS–Automatic Negative Thoughts.

According to Dr. Amen, these melancholy, fatalistic, cognitive distortions can severely limit a person's ability to enjoy life by influencing the way they conduct their affairs, oftentimes alienating others and causing them to isolate themselves.

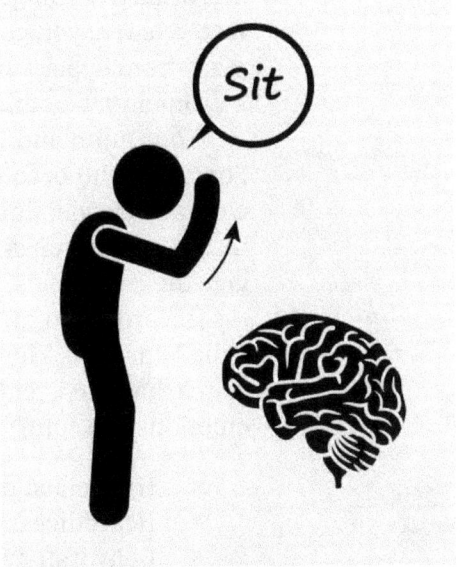

But when a person emanates positive thoughts, radiating a sense of well-being, it encourages people to connect with them. In his mega-bestseller, *Change Your Brain, Change Your Life*, Dr. Amen brilliantly covers how your brain functions, including the limbic system.

With knowledge and practice, you can learn to control your thoughts and change your brain, lifting you to another level of feeling good about yourself because of this new-found knowledge.

HMMM... I MISSED THE CLASS ON CONTROLLING MY BRAIN

There's no formal school that teaches us to think about our thoughts or dare to challenge them... even though they are always with us. People normally see them as random, not realizing they are real, with actual physical properties, and that all thoughts, good or bad, have an impact on each cell in our body when they send an electrical impulse through our brain. Ongoing negative thoughts can overload our brain, particularly the limbic system, by causing us to experience depression, irritability, moodiness, and unhappiness... in other words, not a nice person who people want to be around.

Think of how your body physically reacts when you are sad or angry. You get tense, your heart rate goes up, your face gets red, you get sweaty hands, and you may even get dizzy from hyperventilating.

But aren't emotions all in your mind?

Your mind and body are a team that work in tandem. Someone who becomes extremely upset can experience a cardiac episode. Emotions can exacerbate diabetes, asthma, IBS, and even skin reactions. They are powerful. They give the commands.

According to an article by Kristina Robb-Dover published in FHA, The National Institute of Mental Health states that persistent, chronic levels of stress and negative emotions can contribute to:

- High blood pressure
- Heart disease
- Dehydration

- Insomnia
- Compromised immune system
- Diabetes
- Digestive issues

Negative emotions trigger your brain to release chemicals that make you feel bad all over. Many scientific studies have been done that prove this correlation. Lie detector tests work by detecting and measuring these physical changes you have little control over when you get nervous or upset, like when you lie.

The opposite happens when you have positive thoughts that make you feel happy. Only, instead of getting your limbic system heated up, they cool it down. Consequently, your muscles relax, you breathe slower, and your heart rate slows as you calm down. You feel good. Do you find yourself relaxing just reading about it?

You may not be able to control the physical reactions you experience in response to your thoughts, but what you can control is your thoughts. The idea of controlling random thoughts is foreign and surprising to most people.

Even more surprising is–YOU. CAN. CHANGE. YOUR. BRAIN... resulting in a happier life.

Yes, little old you can actually change your brain... this amazing computer... by learning how to retrain it.

SIT BRAIN. ROLL OVER. STAY. GOOD BRAIN.

The good news is, you can slam the door in Nagatha's face (along with her debilitating, dark, foreboding thoughts) by reprogramming your brain–that magnificent computer. You are the keeper of your brain, after all, the one in control. The only one, in fact, who can train your brain *to think independently of other encroaching thoughts*. You are the only one who can vaporize the depleting thoughts and replace them with positive, motivating, kick-some-serious-butt-thinking that will rev up your motor. The steps below will teach you how to retrain your brain. Permanently! Not temporarily. This isn't a fluffy feel-good Band-Aid.

Like learning martial arts, retraining your brain takes time, practice, repetition, persistence, and building mental muscle. The more you practice thinking realistic thoughts, the more mental muscle you'll build, and the closer you will be to delivering that final kick that wins you the black belt, which is kicking Nagatha out the door and locking it!

It's Cognitive Behavioral Therapy (CBT), the method used by many mental health therapists to create helpful changes in your brain that don't require brain surgery or medication. It's a form of mental health conditioning that anyone can do. By teaching your brain to convert hurtful thoughts and behavior patterns to positive, productive ones, CBT creates significant, long-lasting positive changes in people who struggle with destructive, painful thoughts. As an RN, I worked with therapists who achieved great results using this method. However, there are multiple books available on the subject, so depending on your level of NLMS, it's feasible that you can learn CBT on your own.

Studies repeatedly show the effectiveness of Cognitive Behavioral Therapy:

- Measurable physical changes in the brain
- Changes in dysfunctions of the nervous system

Amy Morin, a LCSW, mental strength trainer, and best-selling author, reports that neuroimaging shows that CBT modifies neural circuits involved in the regulation of negative emotions.

BUT I'M NOT A THERAPIST! HOW CAN I CHANGE MY BRAIN?

We used to believe that the brain we were born with was the one we were stuck with. Some people were born with all the smarts while others were in the wrong line when God handed them out. You couldn't do anything about it, so you just had to deal with what you were given. Many people are still of this mindset, but nothing could be further from the truth.

Improved technology in neuroscience has discovered that our brains are pliable–receptive to daily things we do that can change their structure and chemistry. We now understand that the brain possesses the remarkable capacity to reorganize pathways, create new connections, and in some cases... even create new neurons. The concept is called neuroplasticity–aka brain plasticity.

More *extremely* good news for the NLMS crowd (it just keeps coming), we are not stuck after all! We just have to learn how to facilitate our brains to make these changes, which can change *our lives*.

In his book, *Brainlock*, Dr. Jeffrey Schwartz, a neuropsychiatrist at UCLA, describes brain plasticity–the brain's ability to change and adapt–and his approach to treating people with conditions such as obsessive-compulsive disorders. The steps he uses in his method teaches them to rewire their brains by *changing the way they think*. According to experts, this method of retraining the brain can turn negative and debilitating thoughts into positive, helpful ones. It is also effective in helping people with other disorders prompted by mental rigidity, including anxiety-driven NLMS. Imagine what can be done with your mind when it isn't all locked up and rigid, resisting change.

And I'm just finding this out now?
Better late than never!
Enlighten me.

"HEALTHY BRAIN, HAPPY THOUGHTS."

STEPS TO REWIRE YOUR BRAIN – PERMANENTLY

These are the techniques used by professional therapists to retrain your brain that you can use, too. Research shows that developing these habits can be effective in permanently rewiring your brain, changing the way you think, and living a socially fulfilled and happy life. Dr. Daniel Amen said it best in the title of his best-selling book, *Change Your Brain, Change Your Life*.

(NOTE: Keeping your brain in good shape with exercise and a healthy diet has been shown to enhance the results of these techniques.)

NONE OF THIS WILL HAPPEN UNTIL...

***YOU START LOVING YOURSELF AND
SEE YOURSELF AS WORTHY***

1. REFRAME

Looking at things with *a new perspective* (Flipping Your Selfie) can result in drastically different responses to unwanted thoughts. When Nagatha tells you things like, "Nobody wants you here. See, they won't even talk to you," you can reframe these thoughts with more realistic ones like, "My friends didn't see me come in. I'll go and say hello." Negative predictions and assumptions tend to turn into self-fulfilling prophesies that, when exaggerated, can paralyze you and keep you from moving forward with positive actions. Reframe your way to reality.

2. RELABEL

You must train yourself to clearly recognize unwanted, hurtful thoughts, then relabel them as "false messages" or "brain farts" (my personal fav). Do you love that? Your brain is misfiring... shooting stinky brain farts! Cause that's what they are... stinky. You must clearly recognize and firmly identify what is real and what isn't. Refuse to be tricked by Nagatha, who is sabotaging your own thoughts. Respond to these thoughts by telling yourself (out loud if possible), "These are lies that Nagatha is putting in my head AGAIN to control me." Replace crippling thoughts like, "I don't belong here because I don't fit in, so I'm going home where it's safe," (safe meaning straight to Nagatha's waiting arms) with realistic, encouraging thoughts like, "I'm so happy I came. I can't wait to get

Recognizing our own achievements and strengths is much more powerful than any outside validation. Studies show that writing down and recognizing our accomplishments, no matter how small, actually creates activity in the reward circuitry of our brains.

—Brian Lee, Chief of Product Management at Lifehack

> Stop frustrating yourself by trying to change other people. Start changing yourself.
>
> —Arvey

to know people, make some new friends, and have a great time." YOU are the author of your thoughts, and YOU validate or rebut them by the way you respond. Because you and your thoughts are separate from each other, they don't control you and can easily be sent on their way.

3. PUT YOUR DETECTIVE HAT ON AND PROVE NAGATHA WRONG

When your brain gives you false messages, what do you do to stop them and prove them wrong? Probably nothing if you believe they're true. Guilty as charged, right? Wrong! Put on your badge 'Detective (insert your name)' and investigate. If Nagatha tells you that nobody is talking to you because they don't like you, question it. "What are the facts? Is there is a reason they wouldn't like me?" The answer is... of course not!

Boldly challenge negative thoughts with possible scenarios. "Maybe they are feeling the same since I didn't speak to them. Not everything is about me!" When she tells you, "They aren't going to hire you," respond with, "Why not? I'm a great candidate with all the qualifications!"

Rarely, if ever, will the evidence support the allegations. Defying them one by one by getting that job and making new friends at that event, retrains your brain. As your self-confidence soars, Nagatha's credibility will sink, building your brain muscle (aka self-esteem), and making it easier, little by little, to ignore her. Take off the "Negative Nagatha Glasses" (NNG) and laugh as you tell yourself, "Nagatha's just up to her old tricks."

4. BOUNCERS

Bouncers are your arsenal, your weapons to fight your critical inner voice. You will keep them with you always, on the ready for when Nagatha tries to rear her head. They are your personal affirmations. As you are retraining your brain, listen to the negative self-shaming messages you've been receiving and reword them as positive affirmations.

Do you call yourself names... beat yourself up? How many times have you called yourself an idiot or a failure? I've done it too many times to count. The difference is that NOW it's a way of laughing at myself, getting a good belly chuckle vs. actually believing that I am an idiot. We all make silly mistakes, and hopefully, that will never change. Laugh at yourself... it's okay to be the butt of your own jokes. We can be pretty funny.

5. FOCUS YOUR RESPONSIVE BEHAVIOR

Now you know. The messages you've been receiving are false and you can *simply refuse* to be misled. You have given yourself permission. But now for the hard part–*changing your behavior*. This is where the real work begins. Replacing the old behavior with the new behavior means creating new behavior patterns and mindsets, which is where the change in brain chemistry happens. You are no longer a prisoner to Nagatha, and your brain is *in control*. You have learned to stand up for yourself, seeing the old hurtful thoughts as nothing more than distractions trying to derail you as you devalue them. They are worthless. Empty, meaningless shells.

As your old way of thinking slowly fades away, titrating down like a drug addiction you know you have to stop, gradually, it becomes less intense, and soon, a distant memory. As you take complete charge of your thoughts and feelings, your faulty brain chemistry will change, creating new and positive behavioral responses. Your brain will begin to work the way it's supposed to work... and soon, for the first time, it will see the happier, real you–the one who likes YOU. Instead of heading home to gloom and doom, buried in a Nagatha cave of depression and despair, you will stay and enjoy the party.

SUMMARY:

The steps to retraining your brain are based on the premise that the enemy cannot be defeated until it is identified and understood. That said, you must be alert enough to perceive negative strikes for what they are, when they happen, and have the energy and stamina to win the battle. To do this, make sure you are eating healthy, exercising, and getting enough rest. Throw in treating yourself with kindness and love. Speaking from personal experience, when I am tired and out of shape, I don't always have the fortitude to successfully defend myself against Nagatha when she slips in the back door and the critical thoughts in my head come rushing in. Stay on top of your game!

THE REWARDS ARE LIFE-CHANGING

FLIP YOUR SELFIE ACTIONS:

This is where the real work begins. Nagatha has been secretly living in your brain for a long time. But now you know you can take the steps to fix her damage and live a happy life.

Like most people, you may have:

- Believed you had to live with the brain you were born with.
- Been ignorant to how your brain has been sabotaged by your critical inner voice.

These exercises are one part of the solution to evicting your self-destructive thoughts. Like any habit, they need to be practiced on a regular basis, and soon, they will replace the bad with the good automatically.

1. Consciously listen for negative thoughts for a few days and write them down, including triggers like where and when they happened. (Or anything else that is relevant.)

    As you practice the following, some will overlap and work together.

2. Practice reframing each one.

Example: I'll never get picked for the team! = There's a lot of people trying out. If I don't make it this time, I'll try again next time.

3. Practice relabeling each one.

    Example: You are an idiot. = That's just Nagatha trying to put me down. I'm smart and proud of myself.

4. Practice investigating.

    Example: Did you see how he ignored you? = I noticed Jamie was busy setting up the agenda. He'll be happy to see me after the meeting when he has more time.

5. Turn these thoughts into bouncers.

    Example: I'm good at a lot of things, but nobody is great at all things.

6. Think of how you could respond to the negative thoughts in a self-defeating way (or have in the past), and how you can respond now in a positive way.

    Example: Not trying out for the team because you believe you'll never make it.

7. What are your thoughts on being able to change your brain?

8. Visit this exercise again in 30 days to track your progress.

14
WHY DO I NEED TO BE LIKED?

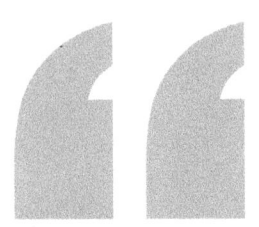

> You wouldn't worry so much
> about what others think of you
> if you realized how seldom
> they do.
>
> - Eleanor Roosevelt

BOUNCER:
Everyone isn't going to like me and that's okay.

"I don't like Joey!" my adorable little six-year-old son boldly announced as he marched into the kitchen one afternoon after school. He looked up at me with arms tightly crossed over his chest and a nasty scowl on his face.

With as much of a straight face as I could muster, I looked at him matter-of-factly and said, "That's okay. Joey probably doesn't like you either."

He looked like he had been slapped and was at a complete loss for words. His big eyes just stared at me, frozen with an unexpected dose of reality.

Seconds later, I explained, "You aren't going to like everyone, and everyone isn't going to like you... and that's okay." You would have thought I had just given him permission to burn down the school, so I quickly continued before his little mind could conjure up that idea... or something worse. "Just be nice to them and get along. You'll have plenty of friends you *will* like who will like you back, some better than others. That's just the way life works."

Sounds easy, right? Tell your critical inner voice that. I believed what I said was true... just not about me. I was convinced that I was different than other people. It took a lot of time, a lot of pain, and a lot of discovery–especially self-discovery–for me to take my own advice and trust that being me was enough.

WELL, GOOD MORNING

You're riding high when you feel you are liked, yee-haw, but falling off the horse when you think you're not, can be agonizing, a real kick in the behind, and a long way down. It can send you into a sinkhole as Nagatha convinces you that you never do anything right, nobody wants to be around you, you'll never get that job, and you are worthless... and YOU allow it.

WHOA–Where did that come from? Well, good morning!

You allow these thoughts to consume you, cripple you, and bury you in self-pity.

Wait a minute. She's the one who said it. I'm not taking the rap for this.

Oh, but you are... for not standing up for yourself. You would stand up for a friend being attacked. Yet you allow Nagatha to beat you up as she sits on her high horse making you believe her lies about you. Who is running this show?

Your mind is probably reeling after that hallelujah call. Does that mean the party is over... your pity party? You're in control. You decide.

Give me a break. I didn't even know she was there!

Great news! Now you do, so what are you going to do about it?

IS THIS WOMAN WACKO?

NO, JUST HAVING A LITTLE FUN ROLE-PLAYING TO HELP YOU BETTER UNDERSTAND WHAT GOES ON INSIDE YOUR MIND.

A friend-mentor-beta reader who read this reacted with a wide-eyed, "That's brutal."

I agree–brutal like your critical inner voice. Fight fire with fire as they say. It's tough love, a wake-up call–and what you do to help those you care about get off the road of self-loathing and misery. It's a splash of cold water in the face for someone you should love the most... YOU. You can get, *"Oh, gee, you poor thing,"* from anybody, especially yourself. Reality can be hard, but it's easier with your eyes wide open.

The only way Nagatha gets in is by you letting her in.

Before you throw this book in the trash, screaming... "I knew it... here we go, blaming me again!" take a deep breath and read on. Maybe she's onto something. Retract the claws because this is not an attack. You've suffered through enough of those with Nagatha–as you know. You don't purposely allow it, but inadvertently, by letting yourself be vulnerable and weak, you leave the door open. But no worries–this is just a battle. Not the war. It's a long way from being over and we're going to close that door. You have a whole life of happiness ahead just waiting for you to jump on board. But leave your old baggage at the station.

> "Love yourself and others will follow."
>
> —Arvey

Nagatha Boot Camp gives you the courage to take the reins by changing your mindset. Get up when you take one on the chin, brush yourself off, get back on the horse, and win. Your feelings are real (the facts are wrong.) They are the result of insecurities... but *I'm really not liked...* and surrendering to the enemy. *Here's my white flag. I give up. You win. I'm a loser.*

Nobody wants to be around a loser. Not even you.

You're listening to a worn reel that's playing over and over in your mind (like the 33 vinyl in Summer of '42... excuse me, but how old do you think I am?) that has to be replaced with new, positive ones. Think of it as casting yourself in a new movie. Is it a horror film where you are the villain? Or an action movie where you are the hero? "Cut" nobody likes me and take "action"... change the script to *I like me just fine. Or I'm the hero that is cheered on who saves the day and is loved.* Whatever you portray yourself as, others will see you that way. That is a commanding action. You set the stage. But you're not acting, it's the real you, not what the false reels in your mind are telling you that you are. Of all the movie categories–drama, thriller, fantasy, mystery, disaster, comedy, action–how do you see yourself? It takes time and effort. I know because I've been there... and I'm not asking you to do anything or go anywhere I haven't been.

A GULP OF TRUTH

Unless you are a nasty monster who purposefully mistreats others–you would probably be in jail at that point–you're NOT the, "Oh, but I am different," exception Nagatha wants you to believe you are. The challenge is to unbelieve the lies you've been indoctrinated with for-ev-er and free yourself from her brainwashing. Can't you see you don't fit in here? You must pull yourself out of the muck that's sucking you back into the darkness with every forward step you try to take to break through the surface into

> "Instead of asking yourself what is wrong with me, ask yourself what is right with me."
>
> —Arvey

a brilliant new light, gulping the fresh air that will heal you and rebuild your self-esteem and self-confidence. A gulp of truth. *Yes, I do belong here.*

Your mission: STOP. ALLOWING. YOURSELF to be a punching bag for Nagatha by getting emotionally caught up in what other people think about you (emotions are transient wisps of nothing). The way you are doesn't mean you stop trying to improve yourself or reach your goals. It means liking yourself along the way. Striving to be better and reaching ongoing goals should never end. When you reach that level of self-acceptance, wherever you are on your journey, the Nagatha-filtered glasses will disappear and you will see reality as you ask, *"Where have you been all my life?"*

DO WE REALLY NEED TO BE LIKED?

Wanting to be liked is positive. It gives us the drive to connect with people. In addition to the chemicals our brain releases that make us feel good when we are liked... or bad when we are not (discussed in the chapter, You Can Change Your Brain), being liked is a fundamental human need. In his book, *The Need to be Liked*, clinical psychologist, Roger Covin, Ph.D., explains that back in the days of the caveman, our need for social acceptance grew out of our desire to physically survive. Building shelter, finding food, and defending ourselves was much easier as a team, but to be accepted by a crew, you had to have a skill that would benefit the group... or be liked by people in the group. Your life literally depended on it.

But what about now that we have technology and opportunities to be social are all around us in our busy day-to-day world? We certainly don't need to depend on each other to forage for food. So, why do we still have an intense need to be liked? The oldest parts of our brain continue to perform the same functions of survival as our forefathers, regulating breathing, responding to possible danger, and processing emotional experiences. In the current world, these also include the risk of social ridicule, financial instability, and even the likelihood of not getting enough likes for our posts on social media.

HERE COMES NEEDY NELLIE!

Hey... over here!

NLMS can make us feel *painfully invisible*, desperate to be noticed and recognized... like I did at the lady's tea I described in the preface. What I perceived as not being noticed equated to not being liked–with the help of Nagatha spurring me on. My selfie was focused on me, which filled the whole frame. Poor, pitiful me. If I flipped it back the other way, I may have noticed clues that would have proved the nagging thoughts (via Nagatha) wrong. I may have realized that the conversations the ladies were engaged in had been initiated *before* I arrived. It was my place to join in. I may have asked myself, "Who do you think you are, the prom queen making her grand entrance to the applause of the room?"

We spend our lives wanting to be recognized by parents, teachers, employers, and others. Always trying to win approval, needing the assurance that we are liked. Even as children, we long for recognition and acceptance from parents (ironically, even bad parents who made you feel unloved). If we don't get it, or even worse, suffer recognition in the way of abuse, we don't feel valued... or our own uniqueness. It's easy to grow up feeling that love and approval is conditional, and that we don't deserve it.

The antidote we seek to ease the pain is confirmation from other people. CONSTANTLY. *When our concern with being approved of by others leads to us being preoccupied with people-pleasing, it's called sociotrophy, a dependency on other people for self-worth.* The opposite of autonomy. It's the salve that takes away the hurting. But it's only temporary without a foundation of self-esteem to support it. A Band-Aid.

Bad experiences can also render us leery of any received as untrustworthy because we have been blinded to the truth. It is hidden by our mask of misperceptions and misguided speculations, like why a text wasn't returned, or why someone didn't speak to us. It's understandable how easy it would be to become obsessed with feeling invisible. Being noticed validates us regardless of how secure we are. It boosts our confidence. Think of how you feel when someone smiles and recognizes you when you enter a room... like the tea. *Hey, you all. Look here. I am liked.* We spend our lives seeking recognition, getting the green light, the thumbs up, desperate for the resulting high we get and dreading the crash when we perceive we don't. Perceive.

NEEDY = LOW SELF-ESTEEM AND LOW SELF-CONFIDENCE

Do you sacrifice the things you want in favor of someone else's choice for you?

Are you worried someone else won't value you if you have a different opinion than theirs?

Most people would like to be free of the need to be liked and approved of by other people, they just don't know how. Their need can become excessive and go beyond normal, acceptable limits. It can become a life-changing addiction, like sociotrophy described above. Their behavior changes. They make desperate self-degrading attempts to make people like them, which many times results in alienating people. Nobody likes to be around needy people who call them obsessively, get angry when not included, compliment them ad nauseum, and wear a sign on their forehead that says:

DESPERATE PEOPLE-PLEASER... WILL WORK FOR A LIKE!

- Are you trying too hard to win the approval of others?

- Are you being yourself? Or a chameleon?

- Are you working too hard to win acceptance?
- Are you agreeable to avoid conflict?
- Are you genuine in your responses? Or are you saying what you think they want to hear?
- Are you afraid of being truthful for fear of being alienated?

I'm a recovered people-pleaser. Even thinking someone didn't like me used to send me into a spiral of self-shame, agonizing over WHY... WHAT was it I said or did? And forget saying no to someone who invited me to go someplace I didn't want to go, or asked me to help with a project I didn't have the interest in or time to do. *What if I say no and they don't like me... or never ask me again?* The voice of Big Mouth Nagatha again. Finally, I realized that being a people-pleaser is a losing battle. If they aren't going to like me because I said no, they didn't like me to begin with. They just needed a body.

Do you inadvertently sacrifice your self-respect to be liked with any of the following:

- Constant efforts to please?
- Doing things that are out of character, wrong, or even dangerous?
- Unwilling to stand alone or go against the group, even if it means allowing things to occur that you know are wrong?
- Agreeing to things that you later regret?
- Becoming hyper-focused on an individual who seems to dislike you, showering them with insincere compliments contrary to your beliefs?

People-pleasers are boring and... obvious. They are transparent and others can see through their charade.

I'd rather have no friends than fake ones

—Anonymous

They come off as fake and untrustworthy, making people suspicious, wondering who's under their mask... or who's going to show up today. They gain nothing except disrespect. Those who are authentic and true to themselves are much more interesting than those spouting self-serving opinions. A person who is genuine attracts real friends because people want to know what they're getting.

- Do things for you, not to impress others.
- *Pursue what you need and want in a way that is wholly you, driven by you, and for you.*
- *When trying to achieve something, ask yourself, who am I doing this for?*
- *Learn to say no.*

Why do you find it so hard to believe you are likable?

To like who you are, stop doing things that make you not like yourself. Things that make you feel guilty or ashamed or keep you awake at night questioning why you did them. Don't sabotage yourself. We derive a sense of self from the mental image our thoughts form of who we are, and it starts during our young, formative years.

LIKE YOURSELF UNAPOLOGETICALLY, 100 PERCENT, WITHOUT MAKING EXCUSES.

THE ONLY PERSON YOU SHOULD CARE ABOUT LIKING YOU IS YOU.

DO THAT AND OTHERS WILL FOLLOW.

But don't throw the proverbial baby out with the bathwater. We all love to impress people with our talents, skills, wit, and our accomplishments. That's normal. (There you go again, being normal.) And it's fun! Life is supposed to be fun. Know the difference between that and trying too hard to be liked. I've spent many hours baking a fresh peach pie to impress a boyfriend or killing myself putting on a dinner party that had to be perfect. It makes you feel good. Who doesn't love the flowing compliments and praises about how talented

> "We are not rejected by others, we reject ourselves ... others just follow suit."
>
> —Arvey

and wonderful you are as you coyly remark it was nothing? Oh, gee whiz. And how about that ex-boyfriend who didn't even notice? Ex being the keyword here. Seriously.

DID YOU EVER WONDER WHY?

- Why is it so important that we are popular?
- Why does it matter if we are asked to the party?
- Why does it throw us into a funk if we don't get chosen for the team?
- Why does it matter if our text isn't returned?

HERE'S WHAT WE KNOW

A positive interaction with others who reciprocate makes us feel good about ourselves. When something makes us feel good, we want more of it. Good or bad, our emotions elicit chemical reactions. Did you know that even the absence of a social connection can trigger the same primal alarms as hunger, thirst, or physical pain (as quoted in the chapter on loneliness by neuroscientist John Cacioppo)? We tend to gauge our self-worth by how many people like us when, amusingly, the ones we are worried about are experiencing the same concerns about themselves. But this thinking is upside down. What should matter first and foremost is how much we like ourselves. That's where the change must take place. All people see the world from their own perspective. Including you. Like the quote above by Eleanor Roosevelt... when you realize that when it comes to other people you're not even on their radar... your self-worth will soar.

WANT TO BE LIKED – DON'T NEED TO BE. KNOW THE DIFFERENCE.

The difference is healthy wanting vs. unhealthy needing. The difference is doing things you like to do and believe in vs. to impress others.

The difference is your happiness and your livelihood depending on it. The difference is being able to tell yourself it's their loss. The difference is... knowing the difference.

FLIP YOUR SELFIE ACTIONS:

1. Do you ever feel invisible around other people, like nobody sees you? How does that make you feel?

2. Did you recognize yourself as needy, a people-pleaser like in the discussion above? What do you find yourself doing that is out of character to win the approval and acceptance of others?

3. Do you find it difficult to genuinely like yourself and be the person you are without a mask?

4. It is okay to 'like' your 'self', this is not the same as inflated self-importance.

    Name five things you like about yourself that benefits others (i.e., I am a good listener).

5. What do you not like about yourself that you can work on (i.e., sometimes I feel jealous of other people's wins)?

6. Do you know the difference between wanting and needing to be liked?

15
IT'S OKAY TO NOT BE LIKED

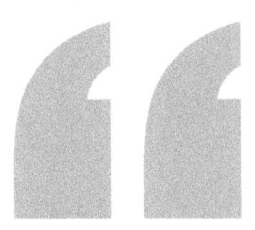

"There is tremendous power in discovering we have a choice. That we are no longer controlled by the agendas of others or our need to be liked."

- Arvey

BOUNCER:
Do I really like them?

THE TRICK THAT CHANGED MY LIFE IN AN INSTANT

You are not going to like everyone, just like everyone is not going to like you.

We are going to get you over that right now by putting the shoe on the other foot.

Several years ago, I was given some advice that literally changed my life in an instant. It's a little trick that may be the best advice I've ever gotten. Hopefully, it will be for you as well. During a casual conversation with my friend, Dr. David Siddens, a clinical psychologist, I was telling him about my obsession with being liked. I told him that whenever I felt like someone didn't like me, I jumped through hoops and changed my behavior. I would do anything to make them like me, including offering insincere compliments, asking for their input when I didn't care about their opinion, and laughing hysterically at their feeble attempts at humor. Dr. Siddens said the next time that happened, I should stop and ask myself, "Do I really like them?" It was like I felt the earth move under my feet. I had never thought about flipping the selfie because I was too focused on why they didn't like me!

I couldn't wait to take his advice. What did I have to lose? They couldn't read my mind... could they? Shortly after that conversation, I put his advice to work and made a powerful discovery. I *didn't* like them. No exceptions. Not even one! Every single time this happened, I realized I didn't like them. Nor did I want them for a friend. The change in me was immediate. By simply changing the focus from what they thought about me to what I thought about them, my care factor did a 180 and enabled me to put myself in charge, put my needs first, and experience a new freedom. It works. Thinking back to the feelings of urgency and depression I lived with all those years, worrying about why someone didn't like me, made me realize how much wasted time I spent being unhappy when Nagatha,

> **"I don't need you to like me to get to where I need to be."**
>
> —Joel Osteen Divine Connection Podcast

> "If about 85% of those you meet like you, you are probably doing something right. In contrast, if much more than 85% of the people you meet like you, you are probably doing too much to get along."
> —Dr. Ben Michaelis, Ph.D.

unknowingly, lived upstairs. *David, the world was a better place with you in it.*

NO MATTER WHAT YOU DO

The reason people are not all going to fall head over heels for you has nothing to do with your likability factor. You will be liked by those you want to like you. Period. You don't need the others. People are going to see you differently depending on their own perspectives, tastes, and qualities. The things one person likes about you are the same things that will make another person not like you. Give yourself permission to be more than okay with that. Be good with it.

It can be disappointing, embarrassing, and frustrating to *think* you like someone when they don't like you back. Have you considered why you care? It took me a few years on the battlefield to realize that if someone doesn't want me... I sure as heck don't want them. It became my mantra, and soon, that of others I coached. The opinions of most people only matter if you care what they think, such as those in your life you value who make you happy, and the people who see you through tough times by reminding you of the wonderful qualities you have. When people don't reciprocate your attempts at friendship... move on. It's your lucky day.

Ask yourself:

"What can I still do if I'm not liked by someone?" The answer is EVERYTHING.

"What difference does it make in my life if someone doesn't like me?" NONE.

IT HAS NOTHING TO DO WITH YOU

It doesn't matter who you are, there will always be people, for reasons you'll never know, who don't like you. It could be how you look, how you dress, how you talk, the way you laugh, your religion, or who you associate with. People will unfollow you on Twitter, unfriend you on Facebook, walk out on your presentations, not answer your texts, trash you to others, ignore you, or not even see you. They'll be offended by something you said or did for reasons you'll never understand. But none of it is about you. It's all about them... maybe something you represent *from somewhere in their life.*

TOUTED INSECURITIES ARE LOOKING FOR A REASON TO BE INSULTED

A happy person who makes jokes may be attractive to some and annoying to unhappy others.

A talented person admired by many may be seen as snobbish or a threat by others who are jealous.

Being straightforward and honest is welcomed by the strong but perceived as rude by the weak.

You may look like an ex from high school or remind them of someone who didn't hire them for the job. I had a college professor I couldn't stand the minute I laid eyes on him. Finally, I realized he reminded me of someone I had a bad experience with in a former life. They could have been brothers.

My daughter approached a good-looking guy in a bar when out with friends and started playfully pounding on his chest, yelling, "Do you know who you look like? My ex-boyfriend." They've been married for twenty years and have two teenagers. They don't all turn out badly.

Most of the time, it has nothing to do with you. They not only dislike you, but you are insignificant in the scope of their world. You may just be something to kick.

They may be having a bad day... or week.

They may be distracted and want to get back to a situation.

- They may be hungry or fighting a headache.

- They may be in the middle of a conversation with someone else about something that doesn't involve you.
- They may be suffering from a hangover.

It could also be that you just don't click. Look at it as a positive.

How is it a good thing when someone doesn't like me?

There is a saying in sales. You need to get nine no's for each yes. When someone doesn't like you (yeehaw)... it moves you closer to someone who does.

In his blog, James Altucher writes, *"No matter who you are, no matter what you do, no matter who your audience is: 30 percent will love it, 30 percent will hate it, and 30 percent won't care. Stick with the people who like you and don't waste time on the rest. Life will be better that way."*

RECOGNIZE WHEN IT'S JUST NOT A FIT

My dad had a saying that has saved me a lot of time and grief. We were both fighters... to the end. Even when the proverbial dog was dead, we would give it one more nudge. He used to tell me, "Sometimes you just have to take your kick in the ass and go home." One of the best pieces of advice I ever got. I had to learn to recognize when it was more about *the challenge* to make someone like me... than actually caring if they did.

Case in point: I'm a power walker. For months, I noticed a neighbor woman walking in the morning. She seemed to be a private (or shy) person. Other than a timid, "Good morning," as we passed, she walked with her (low self-esteem?) head down (naval gazing) and kept to herself, unlike yours truly who even gives the neighborhood dogs a cheery, "Good morning." One day, I slowed down to introduce myself and she responded with a guarded smile. A couple of times later, when I saw her, I suggested we have a cup of coffee. Her response, "I don't drink coffee... but I

"I don't have to have you to be what I want to be."

—Arvey

drink soda." Was that an opening? Soon, we agreed to meet for lunch. Walking to our cars after lunch, I ventured into suggesting we do it again sometime–which didn't elicit cartwheels, but hey, she didn't say no. *This one just takes a little longer to warm up, I thought.* But later, when I ran into her in the grocery store and asked about another lunch date, she smiled, and as she walked away, told me she didn't have time. She meant we just weren't a good fit. I felt it as well, but being me... I just wanted to make sure that dog was dead. My gut was right all along. Looking back, I should have taken the advice of Dr. Siddens and asked myself, "Do I really like her?" Could have saved a few bucks on lunch.

> ***WHAT IF YOU COULD BE LIKED TOO MUCH?***
>
> ***AS IN TOO MUCH? YOU'VE GOT TO BE KIDDING!***
>
> ***ISN'T THAT LIKE TOO MUCH ICE CREAM?***

WHAT IF THEY DID?

What would it mean if everyone liked you? You might want to question which one of you they like... because if you're being the *real* you, that's almost impossible. Even Jesus, MLK, and Mother Theresa didn't achieve that. But why are they so memorable? What did these people have in common that made them so respected that they all hold a significant place in history?

They lived their truth, their mission. Doing so made them exceptional regardless of who didn't like them for being who they were. They held fast to their priorities and never betrayed what was most important to them or allowed the possible disapproval of people like you or me to stop them from doing what was right in their heart. Those opinions would be gone and forgotten in the next breath. How different would their stories have turned out if they had given up on their mission, not lived their truth? This

> "The very qualities that make you likable to one person are the exact same qualities that will make you unlikable to another person."
> —Roger Covin, Ph.D.

is a powerful lesson we can learn from. Stay your course. *Be real and true to yourself.* Reject the urge to change who you are based on the company you're surrounded by at the moment. Don't be a social chameleon. It's an exhausting way to live that destroys your credibility. Nobody will know who you really are, what you stand for, or whether they can trust you. Being respectable may not always make you likable, but it will make you memorable.

WE HIDE

Chameleons are known for their ability to involuntarily change colors to protect themselves by blending in. People can do the same, which makes understanding them more complicated. Their insecurities about who they are lead them to change on cue, hiding their true selves (who they fear will not be acceptable) as they frantically try to belong... somewhere. Ironically, the greatest fear of those who fiercely seek validation to battle their own insecurities, is honesty. All of us are multi-faceted, diamonds in the so-called rough, with many sides that sparkle when we are in the spotlight, basking in high self-esteem and self-love, which is where we aspire to be–comfortably wearing our esteem and confidence for all to see.

Our many facets make us the unique... yet complicated... people we are. They represent our differences–our likes, dislikes, personalities, lifestyles, opinions, views, tastes, and the list goes on forever.

THERE'S A LOT TO LEARN FROM OTHER PEOPLE

People are fascinating. Instead of comparing yourself to others and being intimidated, turn your selfie around... look for opportunities to broaden your insight about people... and yourself. Sometimes I get great fashion ideas, hear about new places or creative ideas, or pick up conversational tips just by listening. Instead of allowing myself to feel like less of a person, I get excited about the possibilities in my own life and ask, "What's stopping you from following your own dreams?" Susie Humphries, a hilarious speaker I heard at a conference, talked about out-of-the-box job opportunities she had encountered during her life. No matter how far-fetched they were, her immediate response was always, "I can do that!" After the first few, the audience would chime in, "I can do that!" The life stories of people about where they came from and how they got where they are, remind me of Susie. If we choose that way of looking at others instead of being intimidated, we flip our selfie and the world becomes our oyster.

People around you share the same insecurities. They compare themselves to you and wish they could be more like you... the way you look or enter a room with confidence, maybe looking at you for inspiration. This is an *ohhhh, I never thought of that moment.* You have a lot to offer regardless of where you are in life. Have you looked in the mirror? When you love yourself, you welcome opportunities to love others and what you can learn from them. You can never give or get enough inspiration from others, no matter where they are in their journey. Be mindful that those you are intimidated by probably have skeletons hiding in their closets just like you.

There was a time when I was obsessed with Twitter and how many followers I had. I had a tremendous number, but others in my group had more. Like those we compare ourselves to, other than their usernames, I didn't know them. I wasted countless hours ignoring important things until, one day, I woke up and realized what I was missing. And the real zinger... when I stopped, nobody missed me. I got in my own lane and stayed there. I reevaluated my priorities, moved myself to the top, and found something interesting. Me. By focusing on self-love and self-compassion rather than trying to get others to love you, you build self-esteem and break co-dependent patterns so you can

"The reason we struggle with insecurity is because we compare our behind-the-scenes to everyone else's highlight reel."

—Steve Furtick

> "Instead of making decisions based on what others will approve of, start making them based on what's right for you."
>
> —Ilene Strauss Cohen, Ph.D., Psychotherapist & Professor in Psychology Today

form healthier, happier relationships... with yourself and others.

STAY IN YOUR OWN LANE WITH YOUR EYE ON YOUR DESTINATION! You don't need to impress anyone with a title or numbers. Focus on being the person you are proud to be. You are the only one you can control. Trying to control what others think and do is an exercise in futility. IT'S A CHOICE! *Choose* who you like and don't like.

What are you missing with an obsession to seek everyone's approval? YOU! You may want to be, but you don't need to be liked by everyone. There are a lot of people out there. If you have a couple of friends, count your blessings. In my many years of working with people, I discovered that people don't change. If they're a problem in the beginning, they'll be a problem up to the end. It's your choice if you want that problem to end now or later. That depends on how much you respect yourself. You are a perfect closed circle that God created all by yourself. You don't need anyone else. What a blessing. I have a philosophy... if someone doesn't want me, I sure as heck don't want them. Choose you.

One of my favorite words is... NEXT!

Wanting to be liked, which can be a good thing, is not the same as needing to be liked, which can backfire. Kurt Smith, Psy.D., LMFT, LPCC, AFC writes in "Psych-Central" that people striving hard to be liked may come across as trying too hard to be nice.

FLIP YOUR SELFIE ACTIONS:

1. Write about your expectations about being liked, keeping the quote above from Dr. Covin in mind if you meet those expectations, and how they make you feel.

i.e., I want everyone to like me but feel I'm at 50 percent. It's upsetting.

i.e., I get it. If everyone likes me, maybe I'm trying too hard and not being true to who I am.

2. Learn to say no to people without guilt. You don't owe anyone anything, including an explanation. When asked to do something you don't want to do, practice responding with something like, "No, thank you, but I appreciate you thinking of me," which is sufficient.

3. When you find yourself trying too hard to win the approval of someone or make them like you, start asking yourself, "Do I like them?" Tracking when this happens will make it a habit.

16
I JUST WANT TO BE ONE OF THE GUYS

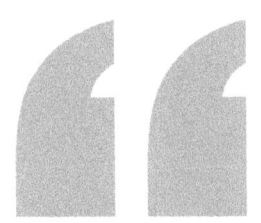

> If you are always trying to be normal, you will never know how amazing you can be.
>
> - Maya Angelou

BOUNCER:

Define normal.

SO, YOU WANT TO BE NORMAL

Why? I mean, normal is so... well... normal.

Do you just want to be normal like other people?

Look at all of them having a great time with all their friends. Why can't I be normal?

But do you ever ask yourself... what's normal?

No time like the present. Take a few minutes and write your definition of normal, as in the normal people you want to be like.

NORMAL?

It depends on who you ask. Ten people will get you ten different answers. Normal what? Normal way to live? Normal way to dress? Normal way to raise kids? The same is true of words like PERFECT or CRAZY. Your perfect mate is probably not the perfect mate for others. You may think some people are CRAZY to want the mate they describe as perfect. It's all about perception.

ONE MAN'S PERFECT IS ANOTHER MAN'S CRAZY. DOES THAT SOUND CRAZY?

SO GLAD YOU ASKED.
LET ME EXPLAIN.

There's usually a laugh somewhere, even at times when you would cry if it wasn't so funny. Like in this crazy moment. When I was a home health nurse, I had a sweet little lady who had Alzheimer's. She was the kind of person who calls you dear with the warmest smile and eyes

"In psychology, normal really means average or typical, but we too easily think if it as a synonym for how everyone is supposed to think and feel."

Jim Kozubek, February 22, 2018, in Scientific American.

that tell a thousand stories when they crinkle. Mary found her way out of the house and wandered off, falling and breaking her hip. As I was doing the paperwork in her living room, her husband, a huffy, broad-chested, former drill sergeant with a silver flat-top and choppy commanding voice sat close by. Mary looked at me from the couch and said, "What's your name?" After my answer, she immediately asked, "Where are you from?" I answered her, and in less than two minutes, she asked me the same questions. I understood that in her Alzheimer's mind, she was asking for the first time, so I patiently answered her again. A couple of minutes later, she started to ask me the same questions and her drill-sergeant husband intervened and abruptly commanded... "Her name is Arvey... she lives in O'Fallon... and don't ask again!" She looked at me and rolled her eyes while making circles with her finger beside her head, letting me know he was crazy. It was all I could do not to burst out laughing... but it was impossible to stifle a smile. Perception. And perhaps the only question to ask yourself is, "Why isn't your perception the most important one?" It should be the only one that matters to you.

Wikipedia defines normality as: *A behavior that can be normal for an individual (intrapersonal normality) when it is consistent with the most common behavior for that person. Normal is also used to describe individual behavior that conforms to the most common behavior in society known as conformity.*

Definitions of normal vary with person, time, place, and situations, and change with societal standards and social norms. Because normal has been functionally and differentially defined by a vast number of disciplines, there tends not to be one single definition. It is recognized by most as that which contrasts with abnormal behavior. In its simplest form, normal is seen as good as opposed to *abnormal that is bad. Abnormal vs. normal can be stigmatized in society and have social ramifications, including being included or excluded by a wider society.*

Years ago, in the 60s, a British model named Twiggy became an overnight sensation! She was ultra-skinny (thus her name Twiggy). Soon, she became popular in other countries, including France, Japan, and the United States, and was named British Woman of the Year. Women around the globe wanted to look like Twiggy and being excessively thin became the social norm... albeit terribly unhealthy. Although Twiggy graced the cover of many fashion magazines, she went on to a career in acting, Broadway, and TV. Thankfully, a few years later, skinny phased out and women could eat again without guilt. *Norms change.*

Normal in society is determined by the expectations of others–which are based on the current social norm (which, according to the 80/20 rule, is created by 80 percent of normal people just like you and me). We all play a role in what is normal. You don't have to follow the flock... you are part of it.

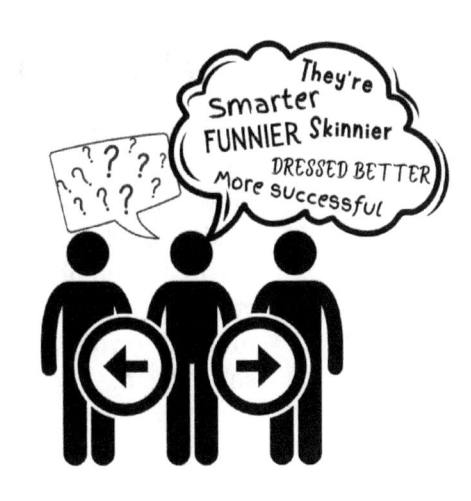

We let the opinions and comments of others filter what we consider to be true. Think about how good it makes you feel when someone gives you a compliment. Because we like to feel good, we make that compliment part of how we see ourselves. Unfortunately, the same is true when we are criticized. By absorbing negative opinions and comments, we sabotage our own integrity and self-worth. We can quickly go from feeling happy with a spring in our step to feeling terrible. By basing our self-worth on the opinion of others, we let them control our self-esteem like a yo-yo! ALLOW–it's a choice. Why do their opinions of normal trump yours? Because you allow it.

If you live your life to please others, you will never be happy. Just like social norms constantly change according to the whims of ordinary people (you and me), your opinions of yourself can quickly change according to the person so generously offering them. What pleases one will displease the next, which can lead to confusion if you are trying to fit the norm of the moment.

ARE YOU SURE YOU WANT TO BE NORMAL... OR DO YOU WANT TO BE YOU?

UNIQUE. EXCITING. REFRESHING.

COMPARING IS DESPAIRING

If you find yourself comparing yourself to others, you have lots of company... it's common. You can't know how well you are doing in school without comparing your grades to other students. And you can't soar to the top to get that promotion at work without being compared to your coworkers. Comparison is a way of life, but you have to use it to your advantage... not as a weapon to sink your self-esteem.

> Must Not Dare to Compare
> To Compare Is to Despair
> And to Others, It's Not Fair
> For Your Beauty Is So Rare

If you're trying to understand why *nobody likes you* or why you don't fit in, you're probably comparing yourself to others in an unhealthy way. Ask yourself what you hope to gain. Are you trying to see how to be normal? Or are you looking for your faults and comparing yourself to how you look vs. the way they look? For example, do they dress better than you, do they have a better hairstyle, or-or-or? The list is endless. Maybe you're using them as your ruler... are you too fat or skinny, ugly or not pretty enough, as successful or talented, or have as many friends? Thinking like this brings your insecurities front and center and sends your confidence into a nosedive. It won't make you normal. Be your own guide to what you want to be–just you.

Why would you allow Nagatha to inflict that kind of pain on you by using the BS she has planted in your head *about your own nonexistent inadequacies* with her 'just so you know, you are never good enough' brew? Flip your selfie so you can get a better view of reality. Like an old pair of shoes, truth is more comfortable (and fun) than her worn-out *blubberish* (Arvey's *Dictionary–feel free to copy*).

Flip your selfie and leap into normal–where you've always been just one of the guys. It may not be as glamorous as you thought it would be (the old grass is not greener on the other side), but it's real, unlike her world of make-believe.

Social media (the world's most punishing and destructive invention), makes it worse with its *step right up to in-*

security touting, *I'm so wonderful brag, brag* a click away. That's a recipe for self-disaster for those teetering on low self-esteem, confirming what they already knew... I can't compare. Don't hang your self-worth on others and their accomplishments. Stay in your lane where you belong. All that matters is you. You don't have the facts about them, how they got there, or even if they did (successful people don't have to tell you how wonderful they are). If you read real-life stories about the lives of the glamorous... they're not glamorous at all. Certainly not wishing bad on anybody, I was not surprised to read about the bankruptcy and divorce of a well-known celebrity... truth or headlines (I'm still out here, fans.) Stay in your lane. It's a whole new world when you are looking outward instead of inward all the time.

Focus on being the person you are... the one you are extremely proud to be.

STAY IN YOUR OWN LANE WITH YOUR EYE ON YOUR DESTINATION!

BE FAIR TO YOURSELF

Make sure your comparisons are fair. Your Coquilles St. Jacques probably isn't going to compare with Gordon Ramsey's! Unless you are a master chef. But it can be fun and healthy in the right context.

While visiting my daughter, I met a cute young couple who lived down the street. In talking, she told me that her mother was an author. I immediately responded with great enthusiasm that I was also an author. When I asked her mother's name, she said Karen Kingsbury. Comparing myself to this amazing mother who has published over sixty books and frequents the NYT Best Seller list would be self-esteem suicide. Rule number one: compare apples to apples and learn to think... I'm not as good 'yet'... which propels your dream rather than squashing it.

WHY WOULD YOU WANT TO BE LIKE EVERYONE ELSE WHEN YOUR OWN DRUMMER IS SO TALENTED AND ENVIED BY OTHERS?

FLIP YOUR SELFIE ACTIONS:

1. What's your definition of normal and where do you fit in? Describe how you see yourself as being normal.

2. Is that what you want to be? Why? To fit in, have more fun...?

3. Ask five people you know for their definition of a normal person. You may be surprised. To make it even more fun, find people from different groups, ages, jobs, etc. That will give you a clearer understanding of the perception of normal.

4. Have you thought about why you compare yourself to others? What are some examples of your results?

5 Do you compare yourself to others to criticize yourself? Or learn?

17
LOVING YOURSELF ISN'T GOOD IT'S GREAT

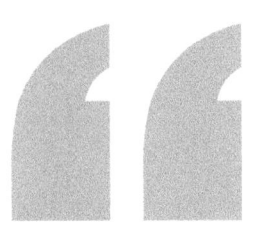

Love yourself first and everything else will fall into line. You really have to love yourself to get anything done in this world.

- Lucille Ball

BOUNCER:

I'm going to treat me like I love me... because I do.

Me: Why don't you love yourself?

You: Good question... it's kind of weird. Not comfortable thinking about it.

Me: Would you love yourself if it could change your life for the better?

You: Really? I've never seen it that way...

Me: Let's talk about it.

PEOPLE CAN BE BRUTAL TO THEMSELVES, ESPECIALLY WOMEN...

I DON'T DESERVE TO BE LOVED IS ONE OF THE MOST DAMAGING BELIEFS WE CAN HAVE.

Why can the most difficult person to love be... you? Think about how insane that is. We say things to ourselves that we wouldn't say to a friend. At least not one we want to keep. We can be just awful–subjecting ourselves to unhealthy relationships, toxic substances, and even mutilation. We even criticize everything we do, the way we dress, the way we look, and we compare ourselves to others who we *think* are smarter, funnier, wittier, thinner, more successful... and Heaven forbid, they even have friends. Would it surprise you to know that those same people you aspire to be like probably feel the same about you?

REALLY... SOMEONE WANTS TO BE LIKE ME?

Why not? You're pretty awesome even if you don't see it... yet.

Loving yourself is one of the most important things you can do for yourself, so why is it one of the hardest things you'll ever do? In a word... Nagatha! The self-incriminating voice of your dark inner self.

> How dare you like yourself? Have you looked in the mirror?
>
> You certainly don't deserve it. And of course, you know it's not polite.
>
> You should feel guilty. Shame on you. Now go to your room where you belong and hide before you embarrass yourself.

As frightening as it may be, your own brain is lying to you with all those scolding, criticizing, ridiculing lies. Not only do you deserve it, but you are supposed to. It's normal and healthy. Stop waiting for perfect to show up at your door one day and deliver happy, all wrapped up in a beautiful package with a big red bow. Loving you doesn't mean you think you are perfect–but then again, define perfect. Perfection isn't a prerequisite to being loved by others and certainly shouldn't be a requirement for us to love ourselves. The only thing required is self-acceptance and forgiveness, and it's up to you to give yourself both (with that big red bow!) And you can do it. We must learn to accept and love our messy selves despite our shortcomings, the same way our friends do.

THIS IS WHO I AM

WHAT YOU SEE WHEN YOU LOOK IN THE MIRROR DEPENDS ON WHOSE MIRROR YOU ARE LOOKING INTO ... YOUR OWN MIRROR THAT LOVES YOU... OR NAGATHA'S.

You've heard that love is a two-way street. But what if it's not? It's gut-wrenching to love someone if they don't love you back. It's one of the MOST mind-crippling feelings. Especially... when it's YOU not loving YOU!

Ask yourself, how can anyone love someone who doesn't love themselves?

> "Most of mankind's misery stems from feeling unloved. During adverse circumstances, people tend to feel that love has been withdrawn and they have been forsaken. This feeling of abandonment is often worse than the adversity itself."
>
> —Sarah Young Jesus Calling August 1

LIKING YOURSELF AND LOVING YOURSELF ARE TWO DIFFERENT THINGS

I have to like AND love myself... BOTH?

Yes, you do. They work together like a squat team to throw Nagatha out the door–the old two-on-one fast-break!

You can probably think of a lot of people you like but don't necessarily love... except in the biblical sense of loving your neighbor, of course. Liking and loving are two different things.

Your work isn't done, but you're doing great. Baby steps. You've learned you're likable, but you now must learn that you're also lovable... and you are. Nagatha's opinion doesn't matter. She doesn't like anybody. You may not be feeling the love–we all have times when we don't feel very lovable... creepy days when we feel a little ornery and let it all go. And who do we take it out on? Someone we love, just like the old song, *you always hurt the one you love*– because you know that real love is unconditional, and you are confident they won't leave. You know if you struck out at someone who didn't love you... they would leave you.

But you strike out at yourself in terrible ways and the only way you can leave is emotionally. You are your own hostage and can't get away. But you can stop hurting–by Flipping Your Selfie and seeing through the cloud of injustices and fake voices that have convinced you that you are not lovable.

Your wounds will heal and go away the second you accept the amazing lovable you, flaws and all, just the way you are, and move yourself to the top of the *People I Love* list. All of us have done things that make us feel nobody could possibly love us. I've spent a lot of my life dragging

NLMS along on that miserable trip. You are not alone. If you didn't have those moments, you should be anointed into sainthood. That's baggage we learn from so we become better people. We all try to be more lovable every day because we will always be under construction.

Loving yourself isn't a destination, it's part of the journey. It isn't perfect and we don't have to love everything about ourselves... at least not every day. Do you feel unworthy of being liked or loved? Don't fall into that trap. It has cost many people the happiness they deserve, including the old me. BN... before Nagatha. Change your thinking. You were created by God who tells us we are worthy. That's all we need to know.

MOVE INTO... "MOST OF THE TIME"

I genuinely love people. *Most of the time.* Blessed to have inherited an outgoing personality that borders on annoying, I had a great role model–my dad. He never met a stranger. Always happy and genuinely fun to be around. *Most of the time.* I even love myself... now. *Most of the time.*

Most of the time is good enough is a mantra I've learned to live with... and even better, love with. It's the *perfect* example of accepting who you are but not needing to be perfect (by whose standards?)... *all the time.* It's a place where you can live in peace with the perfect-less you. One of my favorite *hit the nail on the head, so I'm normal, even okay, OMG other people actually feel the way I do* authors I mentioned in Chapter 12 is Jon Acuff. In his book, *Finish*, which I highly recommend to... well... the world... he makes a wake-up call in his *down-to-earth, this is life* signature style when he says, "Perfectionism is our ultimate villain." Uhhh... yeah! Thank you for reality, Jon.

Isn't that why we are so hard on ourselves... we are seeking perfection? I still find myself trying to do little task-oriented things around the house better and more efficiently, like how I fold the laundry, water the plants, clean the kitchen. A *must be a better way* mentality... or just a little challenge I happen to enjoy. Nobody said we aren't supposed to make everyday mundane things fun!

> "You can't be everyone's perfect. Just love your own."
>
> —Arvey

Years ago, I watched an episode of *20/20* about people who are OCD about perfection. Is that redundant? Whatever they did, it had to be not only perfect, but without mistakes from the *beginning*, or they had to start over. When they made an error while writing a sentence, they were compelled to erase the entire sentence and rewrite it from the beginning. I knew someone near and dear to me who did that, which is what caught my attention. It was like a villain lived in their brain. Then came the saving grace of computers and backspace. But I digress... we are not talking about that kind of *I need a therapist* perfection... are we?

If you struggle with perfectionism, ask yourself why.

Why are you so hard on yourself when a *most of the time* mentality enables you to sit down and enjoy a cup of coffee with your new magazine? Perfection can cripple and even prevent people from loving themselves and achieving their goals. Make a move into *most of the time* and love imperfect you.

SMELL THE FRESH AIR ON THE OTHER SIDE OF PRISON

One of my favorite movies is *The Shawshank Redemption*. If you've seen it, you just got a lump in your throat. If you haven't, grab some popcorn. Sorry about the spoiler. Andy Dufresne, played by the incredible actor, Tim Robbins, was unjustly put into prison for something he didn't do (but should have... editorial side note). Like the prison of self-shame and self-loathing Nagatha has unfairly put our minds in. After years of studying and becoming familiar with the prison, Andy devised a plan to break out by crawling 500 feet through a disgusting, rat-infested sewer tunnel. A small price to pay for a lifetime of happiness. No one will ever forget how they felt watching Andy pour into the stream as he finally escaped his unjustified imprisonment and took his long-awaited first breath of freedom and fresh air. What a moment!

This could be you escaping the ongoing barrage of critical inner voices in your head that have you trapped in your own prison, feeling undeserving of love. Are you being held hostage by looming, self-incriminating walls you feel you can't escape, and voices that fill your mind with punishing thoughts? With the same determination and confidence as Tim Robbins, you have the knowledge to break through those walls of lies and release yourself with a knowing, reacquainting yourself with the real lovable you who has been hidden for too long.

Remember who put you in this prison... people and experiences in your life that have made you feel unworthy and unlovable. The source of your very own Nagatha. You're stuck on a track that has no place to go but around the same loop over and over again, like a toy train in the window of a toy shop, as it continuously plays reruns of her critical destructive voices. Only you have the power to tear down the walls and escape. Once you do, you will discover the real you who has been held hostage for too long. You have nothing to lose and everything to gain. I remember the wonderful feeling of releasing the shackles and feeling the freedom when I finally got it. It was a breath of fresh air.

***IF YOU DON'T PUT YOURSELF FIRST,
NOBODY WILL.***

HOW TO LOVE YOURSELF 101

Do you find it easier to love others than to love yourself? Maybe because that's the way you were taught. Loving yourself isn't selfish.

It's right. It's necessary. It's time. Showing yourself love is also an example for those you love.

"Without self-respect and self-love, we can never be happy when all else goes away ... and it will."

—Arvey

> "Beauty begins the moment you decide to be yourself."
>
> —Coco Channel

Now that you are out of prison, it's time to start treating yourself with TLC, treating yourself with the same respect and love you give to others. Recognize your good qualities. You're a looker, but pat yourself on the back for what's on the inside–your kindness, perseverance, honesty, integrity, generosity, and your caring and gentle heart. Treat yourself for just being you... like you would a friend. After all, you are your own best friend. Love yourself without guilt. Try these examples or add your own:

- Love yourself just the way you are.

- Remind yourself of your strengths and lean into them.

- Take responsibility for who you are, decide which of your messes you want to clean up, and do it without beating yourself up.

- Write down three things every day you are grateful for.

- Embrace your feelings and accept that they are who you are. Help yourself to appropriately direct them while not allowing them to beat you up.

- Routinely have a me date, treating yourself to a spa, hot fudge sundae (that's me), movie, shopping day, hike, or whatever you personally have on your fun things to do list. Go for it!

- Let yourself off the hook for mistakes or imperfections. Treat yourself as the human you are and stop being hard on yourself. Laugh at yourself... I mean, belly laugh, a lot!

- Celebrate successes, both big and small, every day. Throw yourself a party. Stand up for yourself. Show others that you love and respect yourself and expect the same from them. Know your value and communicate it to others. Don't ever back down.

- Write yourself love notes and mail them to yourself. Put self-affirmations around your house where you will surprise yourself when you see them. Sound crazy? You'll forget you put them there and smile when you run into them.

- Don't allow yourself to be around people who abuse you.

- Take time off from the world. Give yourself a me day and do whatever you want. Eat a hot fudge sundae (me again) at 9 am if you want–don't answer the phone, it's a me day. The world won't end.

- Say no! No excuses, no explanations, just, "No, thank you. Thanks for thinking of me."

- Outside of business, avoid life-sucking social media.

- Sleep! Lock the door! Dance! Splurge! Call–don't text–a friend!

DON'T YOU ALREADY FEEL BETTER?
HAVE FUN LOVING YOU!

Give yourself the best gift you could EVER get, wrapped in a big red bow:

PERMISSION TO LOVE YOURSELF

Self-compassion by treating yourself with kindness and empathy may feel strange or uncomfortable if you've never been exposed to kindness or given it to yourself before. Especially if you have a history of feeling unloved or being exposed to abuse, unfairly blamed for issues, or were verbally called out for mistakes.

FLIP YOUR SELFIE ACTIONS:

1. Think about what was instilled in you by your parents/caregivers about how you should feel about yourself. I was told it was unacceptable to say or

think nice things about yourself, especially loving yourself. I learned later in life from friends that it was not only permissible, but it's a good thing. What do you remember being taught about loving yourself as a child?

2. Do you feel comfortable acknowledging that you truly love yourself and accept yourself the way you are?

   A. If not, do you feel you can or should get there?

   B. If you do, what do you do to treat yourself with TLC and love?

   C. How important do you think it is to your happiness?

18
THE MANY FACES OF NAGATHA

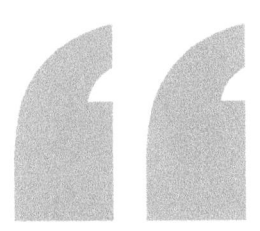

> Don't judge me. You can't handle half of what I've dealt with. There's a reason I do the things I do, there's a reason I am who I am.
>
> - Varha Sharma

BOUNCER:

Who are you to judge me?

Researching and writing Nagatha has enlightened me as a person and an author. It removed *misleading* filters from my perceptions. My mission is for it to do the same for you. Ideas for books or poems just come to you when you are a writer. They pop into your head, and you don't always know how they got there or where they came from. Or the purpose. But there always is a purpose. An inspiration I believe comes from God.

Like most diseases, "Nobody Likes Me Syndrome" is no respecter of class, age, or social status, just like abuse or neglect. But too often, the two go hand in hand.

When I asked people if I could interview them for a book I was writing called Nagatha, I was very candid about the sensitive nature of the subject, allowing them to make an educated decision before accepting. I purposely chose people with a variety of personalities from all walks of life. Nobody turned me down. They all wanted to talk.

I discovered that:

- People are fascinating in the way they cope, survive, and see reality.
- Some wear rose-colored glasses because they need to.
- Every family is dysfunctional in its own ways, but not all are deliberately abusive.
- Normal is relevant.

Is there a common thread or formula for how some escape abuse seemingly unscathed, (at least outwardly for the sake of appearance or survival) while others don't... perhaps by mislabeling it or wearing blinders as they perpetuate denial?

The answers depend on:

- how deeply you dig
- not only how intently you listen, but more so what you hear
- how questions are posed
- how strong your connection is
- the level of trust you can achieve
- and especially, how much patience you have

THE MANY FACES OF NAGATHA

I could have written an entire book filled with these fascinating, some unbelievable, stories of pain, endurance, adapting, and survival. I chose to share two here, and another partially in the chapter called Your Security Guards, that I believe demonstrate Nagatha at her worst, and winning–by evicting her–at its best.

MEET A

Over lunch one day, I had the privilege of interviewing a woman I have known for some time. I was intrigued by her, who she was inside, and was looking forward to the experience. The type of person who appears to lay it all out for all to see, an open book, but you know there is a much deeper, even more fascinating, one buried inside. Perhaps hiding behind something. A protective shield you want to get through. I wasn't disappointed.

A is a very direct, attractive, independent person who can be outspoken. Is known to be. I didn't know what to expect, except I knew it would be interesting.

A was very receptive to talking about herself and her childhood. I was somewhat taken aback by how she opened up immediately. Not only did she not need to be warmed up about discussing her past, but she was also very knowledgeable, personally familiar with the topic of the "Nobody Likes Me Syndrome." As it turns out, there was a reason. Knowing the successful woman she is today, like many, I was stunned to hear her story.

A grew up in an abusive home environment. As she talked, I saw dark. Even felt it like I was there. Growing up, both her mother and aunt showed extraordinary favoritism toward an older sister, while she and the other siblings were physically and mentally abused. A often felt like she was "adopted", a horribly desperate feeling of loneliness and not belonging for a child. And worse, she and her siblings helplessly observed their alcoholic father abusing their older brother. I couldn't imagine the gut-wrenching guilt they endured being powerless to help. Sadly, the brother became a heroin addict and died of an overdose. Accidental?

In our discussion, A adamantly expressed her disdain for the culture of the Midwest "in those days," vehemently blaming it for the passive-aggressive behavior they considered the norm. Her voice vibrated with anger. Not all, but many parents were so absorbed in their own problems, they had little regard, let alone respect, for the feelings of their children... practicing the belief that "children should be seen and not heard." A whipping with a leather belt by a parent was not only acceptable, 'Spare the rod and spoil the child,' but served as an outlet for their frustrations, especially fathers who were seen as the disciplinarian. But not always. Women had frustrations, too. Thus, the passive-aggressive behavior.

Growing up in rural Midwest USA myself, with generations that had lived through wars, the depression, and the hard times of trying to make ends meet and feed their families helped me understand her feelings. Consequently, A, and many like her, grew up with little or no self-esteem or self-confidence–something unheard of and unacceptable in those times. They were of little or no importance... or consequence. Unfortunately, this culture was not confined to the Midwest, or to those times. It is rampant, widespread, and continues behind closed doors even now in homes across the world, not to be shared as dirty laundry beyond those doors. You must wonder if it's something so private and shameful that it shouldn't be shared, why does it continue to happen? It's called mankind.

For many years, A suffered from "Nobody Likes Me Syndrome," often manifesting itself in her outspoken 'defensive' behavior that alienated people. Nagatha had moved in long ago, taking residence upstairs, telling her that nobody liked her, she would never make it, she didn't belong, and that every time she was with others, she would invariably say something that would further isolate them. A didn't even realize that she had an uninvited, unwanted tenant.

Then something happened that changed her life. After years of having a problem getting along with others, being socially ostracized time after time and blaming others, *she recognized that... SHE WAS THE PROBLEM.* It wasn't everyone else after all. But the breakthrough came when she admitted that she needed help. Not only had all the years of both physical and mental abuse shamed her into not loving herself, but she also didn't even like herself for who she was.

As I listened, I hurt for her as she freely shared all the unspeakable things she observed, suffered through, and endured in her life behind those dark and secretive closed doors. From abuse to the helpless, guilt-ridden feelings of losing a brother at the hands of the unthinkable, all intensified by the self-shaming voice of Nagatha, a driving force with the intent of destroying her. Looking at this new woman before me, I was at a loss for words. Finally, I couldn't stand the suspense any longer. I looked at her and quietly asked, "So, how did you evict Nagatha and get rid of the 'Nobody Likes Me Syndrome?'"

She simply said, "I found God and realized that I am worthy."

Powerful. I was speechless... in awe at how peaceful she was. She had put all the bad times she suffered through all of those years behind her. Not forgotten, but over and forgiven.

Sometimes we search for answers, for more, for something to fill the void in our life when it's right there in front of us the whole time.

She realized she was worthy of being liked and loved. If God loved her, what others thought didn't matter. So simple. It was there all the time. She was worthy... a powerful BOUNCER. I find myself using her words often. When I think of her story, I say to myself, "I am worthy."

A is also a follower of Dr. Benjamin Amen and his ANT Therapy that has helped so many, and I thank her for introducing me to him and his wonderful book, Change Your Brain, Change Your Life. Thanks, A, for paying it forward! You know who you are.

MEET B

She's the life of the party and everyone loves her, including me. She has the biggest, most generous heart and is one of a kind. To know her is to love her. The wide-eyed comment by the friend who introduced her to me was, "You don't know ___? Everyone knows ___!"

But something lurks beneath her gorgeous smile, big bright eyes, and incredibly positive attitude. An almost imperceptible protective shield. Almost. Pain.

Interviewing this woman, the queen of jokes and laughter, was jaw-dropping... to hear about the household she grew up in, freely talked about, was surreal. How did she survive?

Her younger sister had a life-threatening health issue at two years old and nearly died. Consequently, her mother became overly vigilant, coddling her, keeping her in a protective bubble with the ever-hovering mantra, "You must be careful."

Perhaps being excessively protective of the baby was the manic side of her mother's later diagnosed bipolar disorder, while her depressed side physically and mentally abused B, severely whipping her and telling her she wasn't good enough, didn't belong, and would never amount to anything.

During these times, her father would stick his head in and say to ignore her mom and not to worry about it.

Her home life was unbearable. She was too embarrassed to bring kids home from school, never knowing what she would find from moment-to-moment, a dark house with her mother in hiding, or a cheery, happy mother.

HOW DID YOU SAVE YOUR SELF-ESTEEM AND EVICT NAGATHA?

At eighteen, B finally realized that her mom was literally crazy, and their house wasn't normal. To escape the abuse, she married a nice guy who was her ticket out of there.

Ironically, her mother's abuse made her stronger and more determined to be successful. She wouldn't give in to believing the lies her mother told her, allowing her mother to become her personal Nagatha, her critical inner voice, in her future.

After her short-lived first marriage, B put herself through school, was the valedictorian, became a nurse,

"No one can make you feel inferior without your consent."

—Eleanor Roosevelt

and married a doctor. Her pampered younger sister works at a grocery store. An all-too-familiar story.

I asked her how she overcame the nightmare she grew up in, and how she saved her self-esteem and evicted Nagatha. Here's what she said:

- I started NOT caring what other people thought about me. They can like me or not like me, and that's okay.
- I always had lots of friends.
- I knew that others did like me.
- I accepted myself the way I am.
- I knew my mom had serious problems and I didn't take it personally.

THEY WON. AND SO CAN YOU.

NAGATHA CAN PRESENT IN MANY WAYS—ALL OF WHICH CAN BE OVERCOME.

So many variables in a person's life determine where they land as an adult, how they overcome challenges, and how they perceive themselves. I interviewed confident, happy people who had the fairy tale childhood and those who didn't. Some had a traumatic childhood, beat Nagatha, and are very successful, happy adults because of a strong role model in their life or various other factors. Dr. Ben Carson, the world-famous neurosurgeon, attributes his success to his mother who told him he was not going to be *a victim* after being left by his father who they discovered had a secret other family and left them in dire living conditions.

My research proved that although our childhood has a powerful impact on our future and who we are, bad or hurtful experiences can be overcome. Throughout our lives, there are many events, people, and scenarios that impact us and build our self-esteem and self-confidence.

They can determine our future, who we are, our success, and happiness, if we don't let ourselves become victims.

FLIP YOUR SELFIE ACTIONS:

1. What's your story? Did you experience an incident, an embattled childhood, or an abusive person?

2. Look at yourself, your strengths, resources, and who you are. How will you implement them in your plan to evict Nagatha and lock the door?

19
HAVE YOU MET YOUR EGO?

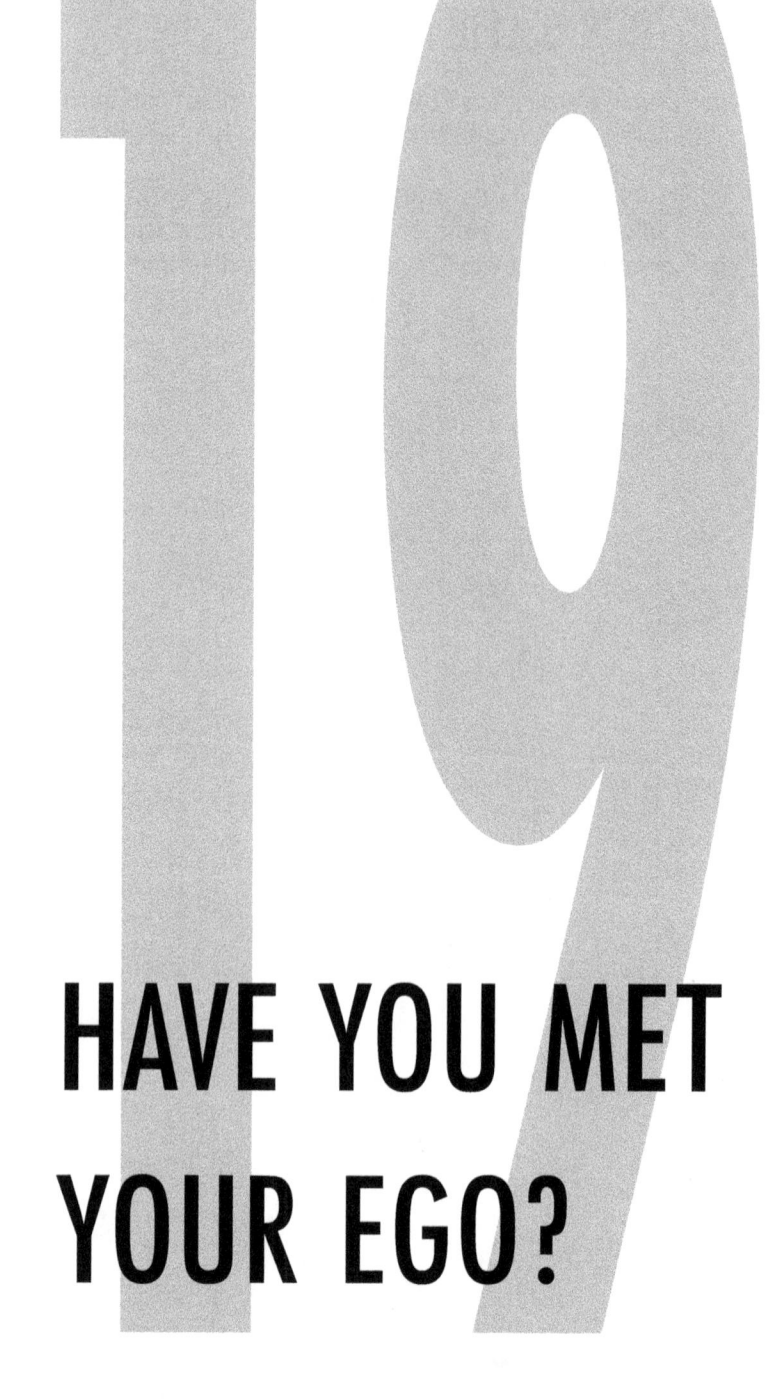

> But enough about me, let's talk about you. What do you think about me?
>
> - CC Bloom in Beaches

BOUNCER:
Is that you or your ego?

Everybody, get naked!

Well, not just yet. Even world-class speakers get nervous when they have to speak in front of people. According to David Greenburg, an award-winning communication skills coach and President and CEO of Simply Speaking, *"Being nervous means you care about giving a good presentation. Your nervousness produces adrenaline, which helps you think faster, speak more fluently, and add the needed enthusiasm to convey your message."* That's great advice for most people, unless you suffer from NLMS.

To quell their nerves, speakers were told to imagine their audience naked. Talking to a room full of nudies would make them feel less vulnerable and empower them, they professed. Fun idea, but it seems they learned the error of their ways and no longer use the naked trick. Seeing nude bodies of all shapes and sizes looking back at them had negative effects. It's very challenging to focus with a total knockout sitting naked right in front of you with that look. Suddenly, your mind goes blank. "Uhhhh... what was I was going to say?"

People with NLMS don't have to be on a stage to be overwhelmed with anxiety. The voices in their head are telling them that wherever they are, people are watching them... and judging. Trying to socialize with just one person let alone a group of people can cause stage fright... minus the stage. Suddenly, they have post-dentist tongue, frozen in place along with their brain as they desperately try to come out with a coherent... uhhhh... anything that won't humiliate them... as Nagatha reminds them that everything they say is stupid.

WHO ARE YOU REALLY SEEING WHEN YOU LOOK AT PEOPLE?

For those paralyzed with NLMS (or anyone who gets tongue-tied when speaking to people), there is another trick to shut down the jaws of anxiety, whether it's talking to one person or a crowd–an understanding of what you're actually seeing when you look at people. Did you know you're at a masquerade party where the magic of a mask makes inhibitions vanish? We used to have an annual adult Halloween party, and not only did we not know who our friends were behind their costumes, but we couldn't recognize them by their new uninhibited behavior. The power of a mask!

So, now, everyone is wearing clothes, but they are also wearing something else... an EGO-the mask master. Instead of walking into a room of naked people, imagine you are walking into a room of egos. But that's not your imagination. You are. And you're packing one too. If that's not enough of a crowd, Nagatha is also vying for her place. It's party time.

MEET YOUR EGO. CUTE, HUH? NOW, WHAT IS IT?

It's fascinating and complicated enough so that even with shelves of books written about it, the ego is still a mystery. We're just going to give you the basics here to empower you to fight Nagatha... and appease your ego.

The English word ego is the Latin word for I... and is included in several terms where I, me, or mine are prominent concerns. The word first crept into the world of psychology via the work of Dr. Freud while defining the parts of the personality, even though, going forward, he never used it. It was a translation of "das ich", which is literally "the I" he used when writing in German.

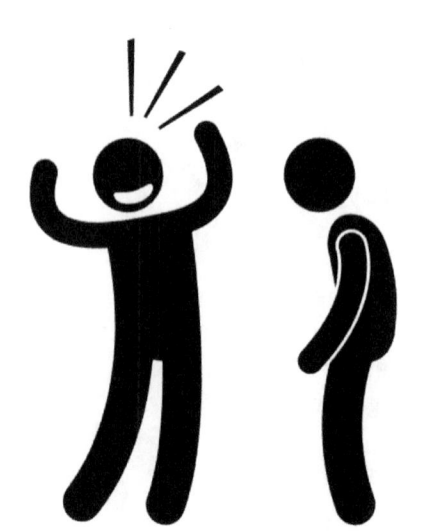

EGOS HAVE GOTTEN A BAD RAP... KINDA

"Hey! Why are you picking on me? I'm on your side!" ...Thanks a lot, your ego

The ego is quick to step up and protect us when our self-esteem is in trouble. It becomes our face. It's the mask others see that prevents them from seeing the real person they're talking to. But be aware that our ego also gives us false confidence. Remember when you put on your Halloween mask and felt invisible... and invincible? The ego thinks it's you. It's delusional, an illusion that can do nothing except be a place to hide behind when necessary. This is where it gets interesting. As much as the ego may come to your aid and appear to be your hero, don't get too enamored just yet. Like your CIV, your ego can be self-destructive by making you feel worthless, lonely, depressed, and insignificant with its tantrums.... yet you still tend to love your bratty children even when they're bad.

Although they are opposites, the ego can disguise itself as your self-esteem and self-confidence. This is much easier to achieve when those two are fragile. Be on the lookout... because when you allow the ego to take over (your 'here I come to save the day' pseudo-hero), bad behavior ensues using our false selves as a defense mechanism to cover up our insecurities.

TOO MUCH OF A GOOD THING

Egos have been known to get a little (perhaps a bit of an understatement) full of themselves, making us the miserable guy to be around by overcompensating for self-doubt with an overbearing sense of pride. "Did you see the size of that guy's ego? It rivals Manhattan!"

And then there are us moms who don't need much of a nudge to allow our egos to step in (moms have earned certain ego privileges).

When my boys were little, I thought every little thing they did or said, and every ornery stunt they pulled (innocently shooting holes in the neighbor's birdhouse with their BB guns... come on, how cute is that?), was adorable. Precious, in fact. I was proud of them. My ego was soaring. I couldn't understand how anyone couldn't see their cuteness blatantly staring them in the face. But my long-time girlfriend didn't always share my opinion. The mother of two girls, she had the nerve to say, "Don't give me that boys will be boys stuff!" after my boys used her newly planted flowers to launch fireworks that accidentally set their field on fire. (Rumor had it that her darling girls were in on it. But

> "The human ego prefers anything, just about anything, to falling, or changing, or dying. The ego is that part of you that loves the status quo - even when it's not working. It attaches to past and present and fears the future."
>
> —Richard Rohr

you didn't hear that from me.) As poetic justice would have it, she now has twin grandsons who happen to be the cutest little boys who ever graced this earth. Precious.

One day, my daughter, a few years older than her brothers, suggested in her matter-of-fact, smart-aleck teenage way, *"Mom, I'm not sure everyone thinks that everything the boys do is as cute as you do!"* An eye-opening slap-in-the-face. A different, and perhaps painfully honest perspective from outside the world of EGO. Mine.

IT CAN GET TOO ATTACHED AND GET IN THE WAY

Have you ever gotten into a heated discussion while defending your opinion about something that didn't matter? You just had to be right. You weren't even passionate about the subject–at least not like you were about winning. Or maybe you've felt wronged by someone, and you became driven to prove to that person just how wrong they were. Our ego thrives because it is an intricate part of us and our ideas, which is why we resent any attempt to make our idea inferior to another, arguing (even insulting), when faced with an opinion other than ours. We will defend our ideas until we ultimately win or metaphorically die trying.

ENOUGH FUN... HERE'S WHAT YOU NEED TO KNOW ABOUT YOUR EGO... FOR NOW

Nagatha (your critical inner voice that exists in the dark side of your inner world), juxtaposes the protective, positive side of what we will refer to below as your ego. Your ego exhibits in the world externally. It's what others see. We learned earlier that our ego is multi-faceted, making it somewhat of an enigma... thus the ongoing topic of many studies. Keep in mind that our inner world of self-talk consists of both a destructive and a positive, protective side. Is it any wonder you are confused? Nagatha is the critical inner voice, juxtapositioned or off-set by a protective, positive internal aspect of ourselves... the ego. Being multi-faceted, the ego is a master at exhibiting different masks to the world depending on how we see and feel about a situation we are in. Both are thought by some professionals, such as Liz Bently, below, to be a part of our ego in their own right, the villain and the hero.

- The ego exists in the external world. Its primary focus is you... and protecting your status and self-worth.

- Your CIV, which is Nagatha, exists in your inner world to erode your self-confidence and self-esteem.

- The battle cry of your ego is, "It's not me, it's them!"

- The battle cry of Nagatha is, "It's not them, it's me!"

- The ego believes we live in a rich vs. poor world where we have to compete to feel good... and only external success will make us happy.

- False identity is its self-defense mechanism, which is what we see when we talk to most people–their ego hard at work doing its job.

- To survive, the ego constantly battles with self-esteem for attention and validation and will sometimes resort to the likes of childish behavior if deprived.

Studies have found that our sometimes-overbearing ego loves us. It's the over-protective child that comes to the defense of a parent. It helps us to:

- Have willpower to get things done
- Stay resilient when problems arise
- Grow as a person

- Become what we want to be
- And it gives us a nudge when we need it

The desirable side of our ego is strong and solid and looks out for us. It gives us a healthy sense of self, characterizing us as valuable in situations where we need confidence and self-reliance (like in business operations). It acts as our offense, running interference, and calling the plays as it:

- Keeps us from suffering.
- Drives our willpower, helping us finish a job, project, or lose weight.
- Keeps us humble, allowing us to apologize... and know when we need to.
- Allows us to be vulnerable, aware of when we are in over our heads.
- Opens our eyes and ears, facilitating us to get the picture and accept–we don't know everything.
- Points out the things we need to learn so we can grow.

According to Liz Bently, founder and president of her own leadership consulting firm, "Ego is our greatest strength and our greatest weakness, it can propel us up, or sabotage us all the way down."

Becoming familiar with the role the ego plays is key in your journey to overcome NLMS by:

- Identifying your hidden insecurities and those of others.
- Giving you the courage to remove your mask and be the wonderful person you are without fear of being disliked and judged.

The ego–something you hate to love and love to hate but can't live without. According to psychologists, they are necessary. Without the ego, we would be mentally ill. So, the next time someone refers to your big ego, you can legitimately boast, "Yeah... that's why I am so mentally healthy."

EGO = ALL ABOUT ME, ME, ME.
ESPECIALLY WHEN YOU ARE A
PARENT WHERE EGOS ARE ALLOWED.

EGOS AND NLMS

Understanding egos is your key to being in control. You can calmly stand back and enjoy the party, the EGO show, with amusement, not judging, but with a smirk of *knowing that says you were there once upon a time not so very long ago*. That was before you joined the, "I control my EGO... it doesn't control me," club, and learned to be happy with who you are, courageously removing your mask and being your new *this-is-me-take-it-or-leave-it-self*. It was before you earned your badge of freedom from NLMS and saw others for who they are, just people with egos... some that were out of control, and some that were kept safely tucked away in a person's pocket in case of an emergency.

E.G.O ➡ *EVERYBODY'S GOT ONE*

People with a healthy self-esteem have unimposing egos (NOT obnoxious), while the egos of those with low self-esteem can be intolerable. You don't determine the size of your ego, people around you do by your actions. You can't always see it yourself, instead, you feel your need to be more than you are. How people measure your ego can define who you are to others, and their impression can impact your likability, your friends, and even your success.

WHO ARE YOU AND WHAT DID YOU DO WITH ME?

The ego has a lot of jobs. It's your representative... your face. Your ego also has to strike a balance on your behalf between the ID (I want it NOW, brat) and the superego (the party pooper morals Gestapo), which are extreme opposites. *Just trying to keep everybody happy right here in reality.* And don't forget, like an overbearing big brother, the job of the ego is to protect you. Tough job. Consequently, the ego's natural state is to live in fear as it continuously looks over your shoulder for threats and other problems that may be dangerous to you. Think of it as your bodyguard... only mind guard.

THE EGO'S NATURAL STATE IS TO LIVE IN FEAR

As the ego becomes the "peacemaker" between the untamed ID and the self-critical superego, it becomes the guardian, always looking for danger, feeling threatened, and the need to become your face... in the face of danger. Your mask. It will always fight for you. Right or wrong. As annoying as it can be, you gotta love that... if you keep it under control. Assume that we all live at some level in a state of perceived fear... a contrived fear that isn't real. Because of this, Nagatha knows that your ego is an easy target... they did grow up together. She is armed and lurking close by, preying on its vulnerability. Her mission is to sabotage your ego. By latching onto the voices in your head, she mimics them as she attacks with her string of lies, putting your ego on the defensive, making it feel like it's not good enough. Thus, the mask. Think about all the self-shaming insults Nagatha throws at you. Target = ego. Always trying to bring it down to her level of misery. This is powerful information for you to understand about egos.

Some believe Nagatha is your ego. She's a busy girl. People only *see* what's on the outside, like a duck that appears to effortlessly float down a creek while paddling like crazy underneath. The ego is a master of disguises. What your ego may be running interference for is hidden behind the mask that Thibault Meurisse refers to in his quote, "Your ego is your self-image created by thought. It's your social mask requiring validation because it lives in fear of losing its sense of identity."

People's thoughts, motives, emotions, and behaviors are infused *with themselves*, with their I. They are thinking about what they want, what they are doing, who they are, what other people think about them, and how things are working for them. Even knowing that, it takes courage to let your hair down and be *take it or leave it...* this is me, but the reward is worth it. When you flip your selfie and start focusing on what you see in others, you will stop obsessing and your life will change. There is no such thing as tidy little *perfect* made of smile and bluster. Perfect is in the eye of the... perfect!

Don't be intimidated.

Don't be fooled.

Don't wish you could be like anyone else.

Why would you when you don't know what's behind their mask?

Just be you.

Nagatha lives in the shadow of your ego, afraid of coming into the light of your consciousness and being discovered. As long as she is an unknown, she is safe and can survive.

Your ego can be your friend or your enemy. You decide.

FLIP YOUR SELFIE ACTIONS:

1. Study what you are seeing when you interact with others. Look for signs of their egos covering for something deeper inside. When you do this, it will change your focus from yourself to them.

2. Get in touch with your ego and what triggers it to become protective. Notice how your behavior changes when you feel intimidated and insecure. Strive to be aware of your ego, remembering that it is on your side. While it is looking out for your best interests, it has to behave.

3. Your self-esteem and confidence hold the reins of your ego. Now that you understand, you have a stronghold against Nagatha. Pay particular attention to how this changes the way you feel around others.

20
DO YOU KNOW YOURSELF? WHAT ARE YOU SEARCHING FOR?

> The world judges me by the decisions I make, never does it see the options I had to choose from.
>
> - Author Unknown

BOUNCER:

Live up to your own expectations.

Do you have the courage to look your full potential in the eye? To see yourself for what you could be, and even more terrifying, live up to it? To follow your dreams?

If you have lived your life trying to make everyone else happy, do you even know who you are and what you want? Stop right now and ask yourself these questions.

Whatever they are, they are your dreams... not mine or your mother's or your best friend's. They are yours. The best part is... you don't have to justify them! You don't need anyone's approval or permission except yours. You have a wealth of untapped potential rumbling around inside of your *what-if* prison, pounding on the walls and frantically trying to get out.

Did you ever feel like you are on the edge of a cliff with your toes hanging over, clinging, desperately ready to launch? You are so ready to just take off and fly that you are teetering, about to fall forward into the wide-open free sky of opportunity–but you are afraid to give yourself a chance. Scared that others won't approve, that you might fail, they might laugh, or you won't live up to expectations, you are paralyzed by *what-ifs*. But are the expectations theirs... or yours? A year from now, theirs won't matter. They will have moved on, but yours will always be with you. Will they be punishing, nagging regrets?

When contemplating going back to school to further my education so I could advance my career, a friend told me, "In two years, you will still be you, with or without that degree. It's your choice and your clock is ticking." Where will you be in a year or two or four?

It's time to fly. As you take off, your own expectations are all that matter as you soar. Those watching laugh in admiration and cheer you on as you follow your dreams.

What are you searching for?

WHO DO YOU SAY YOU ARE?

Do you know the most important person in your life... you?

You're in a bookstore browsing when you come across a book that says EVICTING NAGATHA: *A Journey from Self-Sabotage to Self-Love.* Your heart skips a beat. You glance over both shoulders to see if anyone is watching before you pick it up and glance at the inside cover. What?

You check for dust on the top. Obviously, you are the only one who could possibly need a book like this. Discreetly, you press it against your side as you carry it to the front and glance around before hastily placing it upside down on the counter. Laughing with the clerk like she's your new best friend (distraction), you quickly pay for the book and escape out the front door with your bagged purchase. Upon making it safely to your car, you again look around for anyone you might recognize, then scan the table of contents for the how-to chapter. You suddenly look in the mirror and ask yourself, "Who am I?"

Do you know who you are without all the misconceptions and minus the pernicious adaptations from outside and inside surroundings that can blind you to the real you? Do you know what you believe, your values, and where you stand in the world of life? Or have you been preprogrammed by influences that rendered you incapable of setting your own standards? Peer pressure and media exploit our vulnerabilities and stipulate markers and benchmarks to obtain validity for the purpose of controlling our behavior. If we are not rock-solid in who we are, and firm in our values and how we want to see ourselves, they can coerce us into believe all things self-negative–we are not smart, beautiful, or worthwhile unless we conform to their mindset.

YOUR JOURNEY TO FINDING YOU

Doing an honest self-assessment enables you to discover and accept the real person behind your mask. Its purpose is to help you learn about yourself, not to judge. It's a starting point on your exciting new journey to not only loving yourself, but also liking who you are. And just like my mantra–love yourself and others will follow–if you validate yourself, others will follow. Knowing yourself and understanding your value is essential if you are to function in the world with confidence. Why is it so important?

Awareness and believing your innate worth is critical to your survival and sense of well-being.

There are no right or wrong answers, only honest, soul-searching responses that may touch you emotionally as you go deep to reveal truths you may have buried. Set aside quiet time to think about your responses and allow your mind to drift away from the *culturally-induced markers for validity* we've all been subjected to. In other words, trying to be something you are not, to be accepted. Have fun with creatively playing to your strengths while accepting your weaknesses as opportunities. It's a valuable tool that will open windows as you truly see yourself while revealing how you feel about your worth and inner-most self, enabling you to adjust as you create your own markers. Start by accepting and loving your weaknesses and flaws along with your strengths according to your measurement of self-worth. Your findings will be a treasure that, through acceptance, will bring you peace and happiness.

PURPOSE OF YOUR SELF-ASSESSMENT

- Get to know you and who you are
- Fall in love with what and who you are
- Discover your good qualities and those you feel need a little work
- Recognize yourself as lovable
- Give yourself the gift of freedom

YOUR PERSONAL ASSESSMENT

This is your own work... for your eyes only. Think carefully about each question. Answer each in the way it is most helpful to you. Some answers will be short, but you may want to expound on the answers to other questions. Your goal is to better understand you.

- Are you happy with yourself?

- What, or who, dictates how you feel or act?

- Are your relationships with significant others fulfilling?
- Are your relationships with others fulfilling?
- Do you nurture and enjoy your relationships?
- Do you treat yourself as an important person who deserves the love and respect of others?
- Do you laugh at yourself when you do awkward things or make mistakes?
- What are your expectations of yourself, and do you meet them?
- Are you proud of who you are:
  - Personally?
  - Socially?
  - Professionally?
- What gives you joy?
- What makes you:
  - Sad?
  - Frustrated?
  - Anxious?
- What contributions do you make, and where do you make them?
- Do you feel acknowledged for these contributions?
- Do you feel used, or do you find joy when doing for others?
- How do you feel if people don't acknowledge or thank you for something you did for them?
- Do you think of yourself as a success? Or a failure as a person?
- Do you easily take it personally and feel rejected over things like a friend not texting you back?
- Are you devastated when someone criticizes you?

- Do you have specific goals you've set for yourself?
- Are you achieving those goals?
- Do your activities and lifestyle contribute to your sense of self-worth?
- Are you a perfectionist?
- Can you easily admit it when you make a mistake?
- Do you enjoy spending time with yourself, or do you feel the need to be engaged with others most of the time?
- Do you take responsibility for your actions, or do you find yourself blaming others?
- What are the dos and don'ts, shoulds or shouldn'ts that you live by that meet your conditions of self-worth?
- Are you confident in the decisions you make? Or do you feel the need to seek the reassurance of others?
- How would you measure your self-esteem: the value, respect, and honor you have for yourself on a scale of 0-10?
- How do you feel about yourself? Are you your number one fan? Why or why not?
- Can you write down specific events in your life that were turning points in the way you feel about yourself?
- Have you seriously thought and prioritized the beliefs and values you are committed to? Have you stayed true to them?
- Do you feel that others are better, smarter, more successful, or better looking than you?
- Do you change your appearance, personality, or opinions to be accepted by others?

- Do you have conditions of worth–do's and don'ts, shoulds and shouldn'ts that you live by in order to feel loved, appreciated, and accepted by others?

- How do you feel if you think someone doesn't approve of you or something you did?

- Do you flounder along in blind acceptance of other people's rules? Or are you firm in who you are regardless of other people's opinions?

- Write a description of yourself now and another one of the perfect you. Who do you want to be?

- Add your own questions or thoughts to complete your personal assessment.

Now that you have completed your self-assessment, you should have a clearer understanding of the real you, including your strengths as well as your vulnerable areas. Use your responses as a guide to lead you in the direction you want your life to take as you continue your journey. Include your amazing qualities that make you happy with who you are as well as those you would like to work on. Be your own perfect. Love yourself for who you are because you are worthy and deserving.

Would you take you to lunch? Of course you would.

What better lunch date than you?

If you ask people what they think of you, what would they say?

Doesn't matter. What you would say is what matters.

And that is, "I deserve love."

FLIP YOUR SELFIE ACTIONS:

1. How did you feel doing the self-assessment?

2. Was it helpful?

3. What did you learn about yourself that surprised you?

21
WHY DO I FEEL LONELY?

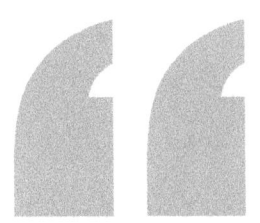

> **All the lonely people. Where do they all come from?**
>
> - The Beatles, Eleanor Rigby

BOUNCER:
Lonely is an emotion—
not a condition.

❝I never knew lonely could break you in two." This tear-jerking line is in one of the thousands, maybe millions of songs written about loneliness. It pretty much sums it up.

If you have "Nobody Likes Me Syndrome"... you may know lonely all too well. They are comrades. You rarely see one without the other. It can be a helpless, desperate feeling you think will never end, like floating in outer space with nothing or nobody to connect to. The effects can be devastating.

But why is it so common? Because people need other people, and there are so many ways to be lonely. There's *stuck-at-home lonely, stay-at-home-mom-I-need-an-adult-to-talk-to lonely, road-weary lonely, lonely when I'm alone lonely, lonely when I'm surrounded by people lonely, I have no friends to talk to lonely, I just lost someone I love lonely, and lonely because I don't know how to not be lonely...* to start with. So, is being lonely normal? Many song writers have made their fortune writing about it because audiences everywhere can relate.

As a home health nurse, I had patients of all ages. I went into their homes and saw how they lived. Had a cup of coffee with them at their kitchen table, laughed, and listened. Sometimes, the most therapeutic reason I was there was... just being there. The visit from their nurse was the highlight of their week. First-hand experience opened my eyes and I understood... *loneliness is a terrible disease!*

MISGUIDED STIGMA

NLMS made me feel disconnected and alone, and Nagatha convinced me that I was lonely because I was different, and nobody wanted to be around me. And even more painful... I thought everyone knew. I would ask myself, "Who knows you are lonely... except you?" I felt like an outcast until I learned that it was my own voice I was hearing–voices that nobody could hear but me. But what others *could* see was how that voice altered my behavior.

Loneliness is misunderstood. Not only do you have to cope with these feelings, you have to worry about being perceived as the person nobody wants to *play with*... or do you? While you will never change the world, you can do the next best thing. You can change the way you look at it.

There is a *misguided* stigma about loneliness, just like there is about NLMS, which is why I never wanted to talk about it. I thought I might as well just wear a sign around my neck that said, "She's a very lonely person, poor thing, because you know... nobody likes her." I was afraid of becoming a statistic... the *'poor lonely thing.'* Nagatha was having a lot of fun stomping on me and filling my head with nonsense once I was down. Looking back to my weak and defenseless days, I realize I *allowed* stigma to drive my thoughts and actions... like it drives the perceptions of others. Stigmas cause people to wear blinders when they don't want to get distracted by a crazy little thing like the truth. They would rather believe what they want to believe instead of facts. It's more fun that way. The truth isn't nearly as exciting as good, hurtful gossip. Identify a stigma for what it is–Nagatha's best friend.

Don't be its victim.

PERCEPTION IS AN ASSUMPTION, NOT A FACT

Ironically, if you are feeling lonely... you are not alone. It's a common feeling, especially for *people-personalities* like me, who crave the adrenaline rush of being around

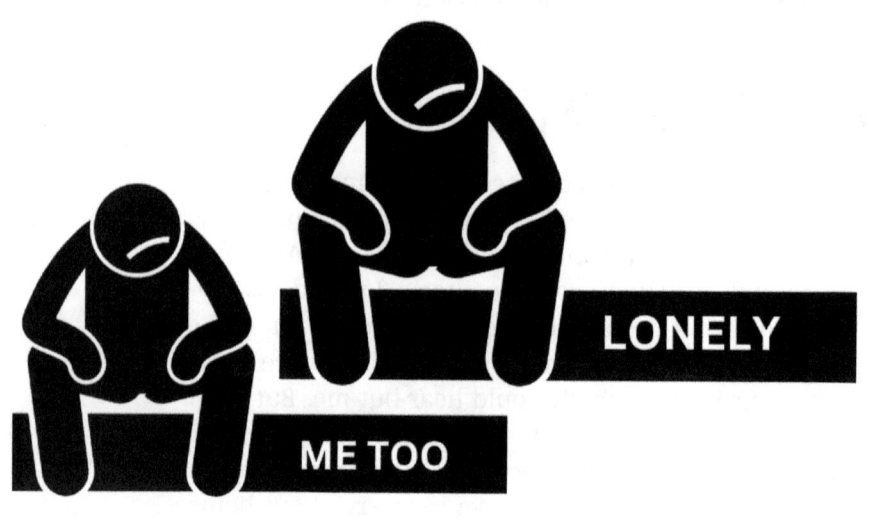

"Loneliness is not caused by others. It's when your mind tells you that Nobody Cares About You."

- QuotesLifeTime.com

people. But that's not everybody. Some, like my granddaughter, prefer traveling to exciting places with friends via the depths of a good book. When a book is your best friend, you're seldom lonely. Different personalities make for an interesting world. To quell your lonely feelings, start by not chiming in with the voices trying to persuade you that being alone is your fault. Then do your homework. Where's the evidence that makes you believe this malarkey? There isn't any! But there is evidence that you are wrong. Struggling with loneliness, or feeling left out, is as common as the common cold. The numbers are staggering, in the millions! Statically, half of those around you are feeling it, but you probably wouldn't recognize them... *the poor lonely things.*

A 2018 Cigna survey of 20,000 adults used the UCLA Loneliness Scale to determine that "Nearly half of Americans report they sometimes or always feel alone (46%) or left out (47%)." They claim loneliness has reached epidemic levels across all age groups.

Sadly, many don't even question why because they have it all figured out–they are just different from other people and *deserve* what they get. Case closed. They judge themselves, blame themselves, shame themselves and believe the nagging voices of their CIV. They have literally been... brainwashed... in the truest sense of the word–by their own brain!

Now that I know that it's my choice, I love my time alone. I can't get enough of it... alone with the new me I've learned to love. Flip your selfie and see the difference. The goal of this book is for you to acquire the self-esteem and confidence you need to combat these misleading voices and evict them. Learn how to exchange feeling lonely for coveting your alone time. That's what you deserve... loving time with you. But beware, it's easy to OD.

WHAT IS LONELINESS?

It's an emotion (feeling), opposed to a condition like a disease, that can change quickly. Like when you suddenly get good news... or bad. We all experience loneliness when a best friend moves away or a relationship ends, for example. The subject is so prevalent in determining the quality of our lives that many scientific studies have been done to determine its cause–how loneliness affects us both physically and psychologically, and how to overcome it.

John Cacioppo, a neuroscientist who has made a career out of studying loneliness, defines it as "Perceived isolation, or the difference between what you want from your social relationships and where you are with those relationships." According to him, the absence of a social connection triggers the same, primal alarm bells as hunger, thirst, and physical pain.

Cacioppo states, "Loneliness is like an iceberg–it goes deeper than we can see." He further explains, "Loneliness is contagious, heritable, and affects one in four people–and increases the chances of early death by 20%." Fortunately, he believes it can be treated.

Contrary to popular belief, it is not about being by yourself. It IS about CONNECTING with anyone you can share things with. Including yourself!

YOURSELF? YES–THAT IS WHERE YOU NEED TO START.

IN THE WAR AGAINST LONELINESS, THE MOST IMPORTANT RELATIONSHIP YOU SHOULD NURTURE FOR YOUR OWN WELL-BEING IS THE CONNECTION WITH YOURSELF.

If you struggle with NLMS, self-disparaging feelings of total separateness can become part of your everyday life. After many years of bad relationships, feeling lonely, beating myself up, and blaming everyone else, I had a head-on come-to-Jesus meeting with the mirror and finally saw what I was missing... a healthy connection with *myself*. Reflecting back, I could see how needy I was, depending on others to fill my emptiness, terrified of being alone. Is that you?

I had to go to my own school to learn how to connect with myself (before I could connect with others), to enjoy my own company, dinner for one, read a good book together–me and me. When I did, it was like a tremendous weight was lifted. No longer dependent on others for fulfillment, I was free as a butterfly. No longer afraid to be alone.

Are you connected with you? The one person you should always be able to count on is you... being there for you. You don't even have to make a date. You are always available. But you have to practice having one-on-one dates with you. It's really okay... even legal and healthy. Like you just discovered smoothies. Start by planning a weekly date with just you... and keep it. You wouldn't cancel on anyone else.

When my husband is out of town, the new me will grab a good book I can bury myself in and go out for dinner. When a young woman in our office overheard me say where I was headed one afternoon, she was horrified. We are talking dropped jaw and wide-eyed surprise. She made the comment, "I could never do that!" When I asked why, she said she would feel too embarrassed to go someplace public by herself. Maybe she was afraid of the stigma of being seen as a "poor, lonely thing." We know who put that in her head... her upstairs roommate. It's really okay, girlfriend, to be your own hot date. Try it. You may not believe it, but... no one is watching.

Laugh off the opinions of others. Stigmas are unfounded. Investigate and form your own educated opinion. That's the only one that matters anyway. You may be surprised to find that poor, lonely soul prefers to be alone. But it's alright to ask. You will never be lonely when you have a healthy connection with yourself. Anyone who judges you for that is a sister of Nagatha. Give her the boot.

CONNECTIONS LEAVE LONELINESS IN THE DUST

If you were asked to draw loneliness, what would you draw?

A person all alone in a room, or at home watching television by themselves? Or maybe someone in a crowd with a sad face whose only connection is Nagatha, telling them they don't belong because nobody wants them there?

What's your loneliness? For some people, a life event or a holiday can trigger it. Or a memory. Yearning for things we lose often manifests itself as loneliness.

SEASONS OF OUR LIFE AMONG MANY OTHER FACTORS CAN CONTRIBUTE TO FEELINGS OF LONELINESS

Like trees that bud in the spring and lose their leaves in the fall, we have seasons in our lives that affect our feelings. According to Dr. Dilip Jest, research suggests that "loneliness severity and age have a complex relationship, with increased loneliness in the late 20s, mid-50s, and late 80s." These ages may be significant with changes in our seasons. "One thing to remember is that loneliness is subjective. Loneliness does not mean being alone; loneliness does not mean not having friends," said Dr. Jeste, who is also director of UC San Diego's Centre for Healthy Ageing. "Loneliness is defined as 'subjective distress'. It is the discrepancy between the social relationships you want and the social relationships you have," he said.

Why we feel lonely is a bit of a mystery and affects everyone differently. What about you? Is your loneliness debilitating? Does it negatively affect your life, your happiness? Does it send you spiraling into a depression that feels like it will never end? There is hope. It's up to you to stop waiting... and take the first step.

WHAT'S THE ANSWER? CONNECT

The common thread to combating loneliness is connecting. But it's not unusual for people to not know HOW to connect, where to go, or how to start. They feel they are loners, the odd one out, unaware there are many others JUST like them, looking to connect with someone who has common interests, who can share like experiences and memories. It's relating with someone, hooking up, and enjoying being together, not judging or being judged or feeling threatened. People tend to think they need many connections, but just one in your life can change your world and mean the difference between being lonely... and not lonely.

Maybe you feel you can't connect with others because you have nothing to offer, are different, or unlikeable, so you don't even try for fear of rejection. Your neighbor could be feeling the same. But there is someone for everyone who is looking for others to reach out to them. No one wants to be alone. A wise man, my dad, taught me, "You never get anything you don't ask for." Is rejection worse than the painful loneliness you are living with now?

NOT JUST CONNECTIONS. HEALTHY CONNECTIONS

Being lonely in a crowd is a helpless, empty feeling fraught with anxiety. It's like teetering on the edge of a cliff, ready to jump with no place to jump to. Your brain silently screams to be rescued. It's a frantic feeling of reaching out to grab onto someone to keep from falling, but there's no one to catch you. It can even be when you are with a life partner or friend but feel no connection. A study done by Cigna shows that even those who live with others are only slightly less likely to be lonely than those who live alone. Like Dr. Jeste said, loneliness isn't about being alone. It's about connections.

An experience I had a few years ago prompted me to write Nagatha. With a heavy heart, my son told me that he and his wife were moving to Nashville—a decision I could have lived with BUT... that meant my four granddaughters who were my world were leaving, too. I was hysterical... verging on being suicidal. After twelve years, I couldn't imagine not seeing them in our pool every other day, attending every school event, every dance recital, and being a part of their daily lives. For weeks, I was curled up in a ball in my pajamas. The pain was more than I could bear. Sobbing uncontrollably, I picked up my phone to call someone, a friend, when I realized I had no one to call. Nobody I could trust to understand, listen, and not judge. With hundreds of friends, including five thousand useless Facebook 'friends', I had no one I felt connected to enough to cry with. I was all alone. It opened my eyes to what I was missing... connections.

Healthy connections give us a sense of value. And happiness. They put a bounce in our step. They make us bubble with energy and give us a spark, like when you're in a spunky, effortless, nothing conversation with a friend. Healthy connections boast self-esteem and the confidence to pursue other healthy connections.

Bad connections do just the opposite. Don't keep people in your life that bring you down just to have someone... get rid of them. There are plenty of others who will lift you up. The standards you adhere to in choosing who you associate with determines who you attract. Desperation can inadvertently cause people with "Nobody Likes Me Syndrome" to make bad decisions. I made a few regretful ones. Don't settle. Hold out for the right healthy connections.

JUMP INTO REALITY AND THROW AWAY THE CRUTCH

Do you agree that *all 47 percent of Americans* who are lonely see themselves as weird, unwanted, undesirable losers, outcasts that others don't want to be around, certain that others see them the same way? If you are pointing to yourself as one of them, put your finger down... you're wrong. There is nothing wrong with you. Those you believe are seeing you that way probably aren't seeing you at all. They don't even know you exist! And that's the problem.

"Courage is not having the strength to go on. It is going on when you don't have the strength."

—Theodore Roosevelt

"I can't reach out, but I'll reach back."

—Arvey

Why don't they know you exist? Is it fear? Fear clouds your thinking. It's not going to get any better until you muster up the courage to confront it.

The first connection is the hardest. It's also your lifeline, your door-buster. It breaks down the wall that's been keeping you hidden away from the scary world you thought was behind it. One successful encounter will seed your confidence and move you forward in a new healthy direction. But you have to take that step. I could drag you around to every place and everyone in town to no avail. You can't get courage through osmosis.

Locking yourself away has much more serious consequences than you could possibly encounter otherwise. Get out there. Find people who share your interests. Reach out and connect. How about a cup of coffee?

FLIP YOUR SELFIE ACTIONS:

1. Describe your loneliness and what triggers it.

    A. Does it have a negative effect on your life?

2. Why do you think you're lonely?

    A. It's my fault, nobody wants to be with me.

    B. I don't have any intimate connections.

    C. I don't feel lonely beyond normal.

    D. Other.

3. Draw loneliness as you see it.

4. Describe the social connections you currently have.

    A. Now describe the ones you want.

    B. Do you feel you have healthy connections?

- C. Does the thought of reaching out to make connections make you fearful?
- D. Will you be the one to reach out? Or reach back? Maybe both.

5. Do you enjoy your time alone? Or do you use it as an excuse to stay in hiding?

22
ISOLATION IS NAGATHA'S BEST FRIEND

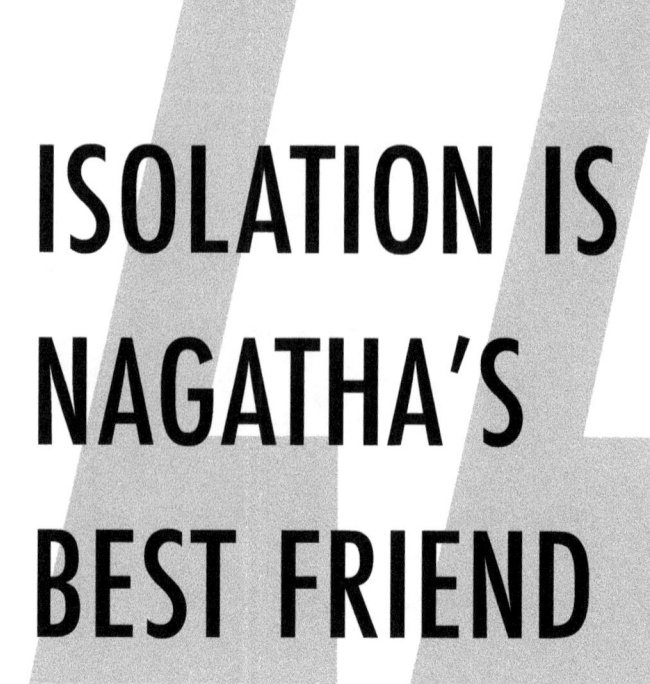

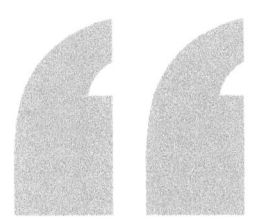

> A season of loneliness and isolation is when the caterpillar gets its wings. Remember that next time you feel alone.
>
> - Mandy Hale

BOUNCER:
Find your wings and take flight. Connect.

PUT ON THE GLOVES

Nerves! Just Nerves!
These three little words caught my attention. Little... but mighty.

Written in bold letters, this was the title of a brochure I saw in a doctor's office a few years ago. *That looks interesting*, I thought as I unfolded it. Even as an RN, I was astonished to discover what our nervous system can do to us. *Where was that hidden in the textbook?* We're not talking about feeling a little jittery about your first day at work or facing those dreaded scales at your doctor's office–we're talking some powerful stuff. Controlling, life-changing, disease-causing, and even fatal! Who would have thought these little spidery-looking neurons scattered throughout our bodies could be so powerful?

Did you ever feel like you were going to pass out, or even worse, wet your pants when you had to walk onto a stage in front of a large group of people and perform? How were you supposed to hit any of the right keys with frozen fingers in those terrifying piano recitals when you were a kid? All those threatening faces staring at you with imagined score cards in their hands waiting to judge you... while your brain was saying... calm down. Just hang in there and fight this quickly approaching meltdown–you can do this.

Or maybe it's screaming...

> ***RUN! JUST GET OUT NOW WHILE YOU CAN! GO HOME AND HIDE SAFELY BEHIND CLOSED DOORS!***

FIGHT OR FLIGHT

We all have a built-in *Fight or Flight* mechanism, an instinctive physiological reaction to a threatening or stressful situation, which readies our sympathetic nervous system to either fight... or run. According to "Understanding the Stress Response," an article in Harvard Health Publishing, *"The Fight-or-Flight response evolved as a survival mechanism, enabling people and other mammals to react quickly* to life-threatening situations. The carefully orchestrated yet near-instantaneous sequence of hormonal changes and physiological responses helps someone to fight the threat off or flee to safety. Unfortunately, the body can also overreact to stressors that are not life-threatening, such as traffic jams, work pressure, and family difficulties."

Those overwhelming feelings you get before playing the piano in that recital or speaking to a group of people are examples of this response. Your nerves take over, you can't breathe, your heart races, your hands are sweaty, and you desperately want to disappear. Quickly.

Much the same as when Nagatha starts doing her dirty work. With NLMS, it's typical to feel that you are on stage any time you are around people, especially in a group. Your evil inner voice fills your head with vicious lies, cleverly mimicking your own voice as it convincingly shames you into believing you need to run. *You know you're going to make a fool of yourself flubbing up that song.* Nagatha engages your flight mechanism, shouting at you to isolate yourself behind closed doors in the comfort of her welcoming arms. *She will protect you from those people who don't like you, and furthermore, never will.* Even though you know you're not in danger, your mind feels threatened and triggers the fight or flight response. You have a choice.

FIGHT OR FLIGHT?

Your gut hurts. Your brain is screaming, 'Choose flight and get away from this agonizing pain! I don't have the energy to fight it anymore. You win. Nobody likes me and I just want to go home. So what if I have to isolate myself to get relief? At least the pain will stop. Just avoid social situations and I'll be safe... right?'

WRONG... DANGEROUSLY WRONG.

THERE'S MORE TO ISOLATION THAN ISOLATION. DON'T RUN INTO THE ARMS OF THE ENEMY.

NLMS ISN'T CONTROLLED BY NAGATHA... IT IS NAGATHA!

> Once you fall in, you tend to go deeper and deeper into the mire. As you slide down those slippery walls, you are well on your way to depression, the darkness is profound.
>
> - Sarah Young, *Jesus Calling* July 16, Psalm 40:2-3

Giving into Nagatha by *allowing* yourself to be forced into isolation as a means of escape is only exacerbating the wounds. Anyone who has ever stopped any self-destructive behavior, i.e., smoking, knows that if you're ever going to get it behind you, you have to get over the hump, sometimes the mountain, whether it's today or five years from now. You must choose fight vs. flight.

We are instinctively social, so it's natural to feel alone when isolated from others. However, when left alone with our thoughts, loneliness can turn up the volume on the soundtrack of our critical inner voice even louder. Isolation is a perfect breeding ground for Nagatha and her self-destructive attacks, making it nearly impossible to defend yourself as she buries you deeper and deeper, encouraging you to avoid others. She has you all to herself in a quiet, secure place you may mistakenly think of as your safe haven, when actually... it's hers.

Isolation is an unhealthy retreat that can be harmful to your health as it leads you into a dangerous place... like the drunk who tried to drown his problems, only to wake up and discover they could swim. There are unimaginable consequences in choosing flight over fight and retreating into isolation. It's a petri dish that feeds and intensifies Nagatha's thoughts and drowns you in your isolated self-pity.

SELF-PITY IS A SLIMY, BOTTOMLESS PIT.

SOLITUDE VS. ISOLATION

Don't confuse them... they are two different things. Solitude is a healthy choice you make because you enjoy the peace and quiet of your own company in a place where you can totally be you. Solitude can be a healthy rejuvenating experience, allowing you to get back in touch with yourself. Some people enjoy and need solitude more than others, especially introverts. A steady diet of social interacting with others can be draining to an introvert. Even extroverts can crave a reprieve from the stimuli of hobnobbing.

- Solitude is the state of being alone.
- Isolation is a lack of social relationships or emotional support.
- Loneliness is a craving for social contact. It means there is discomfort, wanting to be connected to others, and often linked to feelings of sadness and emptiness.

The devastating effects isolation can have on your health are much worse than loneliness.

From personal experience, extreme isolation can have catastrophic effects, both physically and mentally. I am adamant on this subject because I've seen it... it's real. My cousin, a delightful, handsome young man I adored, couldn't cope with the self-destructive thoughts in his head. He isolated himself... and died.

SOCIAL AND EMOTIONAL ISOLATION

Solitude is simply the state of being alone and can be chosen or forced due to a situation, like moving to a new area. It can also be a health choice, such as taking a mental health day.

Social Isolation is the absence of social relationships. While solitude can be welcome, social isolation is unwanted and harmful. It's an escape from a life someone can't cope with. (PLEASE SEE BELOW.)

Emotional Isolation–when a person is unable or unwilling to share their emotions with others–can occur due to social isolation. It can act as a defense mechanism to shield a person from distress. Even with a social network, a person can keep themselves emotionally isolated.

You can see how the two can work together with victims of NLMS, using isolation to protect themselves from the pain of Nagatha's relentless negative thoughts, convincing them they are not socially wanted or acceptable.

You may be experiencing social isolation if you find yourself:

- Avoiding social interaction due to shame or depression.
- Spending extended periods of time alone.
- Experiencing Social Anxiety (see below) or fear of abandonment at the thought of social interaction.
- Having limited or superficial social contact.
- Lacking important social or professional relationships.
- Developing severe distress and loneliness.

SOCIAL ANXIETY DISORDER

After witnessing the calamitous effects Social Isolation can have, I've included a brief discussion here about Social Anxiety, also known as *Social Phobia*–one of the most common mental health illnesses affecting nearly 15 million adults in the US alone. Although lab work or imaging is not required, it must be diagnosed by a healthcare professional. Social Anxiety, where everyday social interactions cause extreme irrational anxiety, is a chronic mental health condition that can last for years, or even a lifetime. While "Nobody Likes Me Syndrome" can share some of the milder symptoms, it should NOT BE CONFUSED WITH SOCIAL ANXIETY DISORDER, which manifests at a whole new level of severity.

This condition is characterized by feelings of *intense anxiety and fear* of being judged by people in social situations, whether the worry is that you won't be liked, or that you'll do something to embarrass yourself. Even seemingly benign personal interactions like those below can cause this irrational anxiety and severe emotional discomfort. It can be so extreme that using a public restroom or eating and drinking in a restaurant causes a person to experience debilitating symptoms.

Social Anxiety can occur when experiencing things such as:

- Meeting new people
- Talking with your boss

- Interacting with a teller at a bank
- Going on a date
- Ordering flowers, even by phone
- Job interviews
- Answering a question in a classroom

People with this disorder feel out of control. It interferes with routine activities like work and school, causing them to often dread any upcoming interaction with people for weeks *ahead of time*. They find themselves making excuses not to attend events, even church or a best friend's wedding, for fear of having to do something that would humiliate or embarrass them. Everyday social interactions can be emotionally crippling from inappropriate situational anxiety and fear, self-consciousness, and embarrassment.

Victims of Social Anxiety will frequently resort to social withdrawal and isolation as a way to escape the agony and frustrations of their daily life–such as a persistent fear of being watched, of being judged, disgraced, and criticized by others. Their feelings of shame, guilt, and worries about offending someone each time they must interact with other people can become overwhelming and insurmountable. As it consumes their lives, Social Anxiety can make it difficult to cultivate and keep friends.

Signs of potential Social Anxiety to be aware of:

- Extremely paranoid of being judged by others.
- Inappropriately self-conscious at everyday social situations.
- Going to extreme measures to avoid meeting new people.
- Experiencing an intense desire to run away.
- Difficulty talking to people at work or school.
- Severe physical symptoms of anxiety, including excessive sweating, rapid breathing, GI pains, or headaches.

If a person suffering from this disorder is not treated, it can lead to even more severe conditions like depression, panic disorder, and complete isolation. The good news is that treatment by a medical professional can help overcome these symptoms.

FLIP YOUR SELFIE ACTIONS:

1. Have you experienced Fight or Flight? For example, running from a situation rather than fighting through it?

   Talk about which you chose, fight or flight. If you had it to do again, would you make the same choice? I can recall times when I've done both. As I matured, I learned that fighting through most of them vs. fleeing had more rewarding outcomes that I was able to learn from. (Never stay in a life-threatening situation!)

2. Do you understand the difference between solitude, isolation, and loneliness, and the value or negative effects of each?

   A. Have you experienced them? If so, think of why and how each affected you.

3. Social Anxiety is not a condition to be taken lightly. It's not something to be ashamed of and it can be treated with professional help, which is confidential. If you find yourself isolating, do an honest self-evaluation of the severity of your reasons and how they are affecting your mental and physical health, and your life.

IF YOU HAVE SYMPTOMS OF SOCIAL ANXIETY OR SUICIDAL THOUGHTS, SEEK PROFESSIONAL HELP!

SAMHSA'S NATIONAL HELPLINE – 1-800-662-HELP (4357)

23

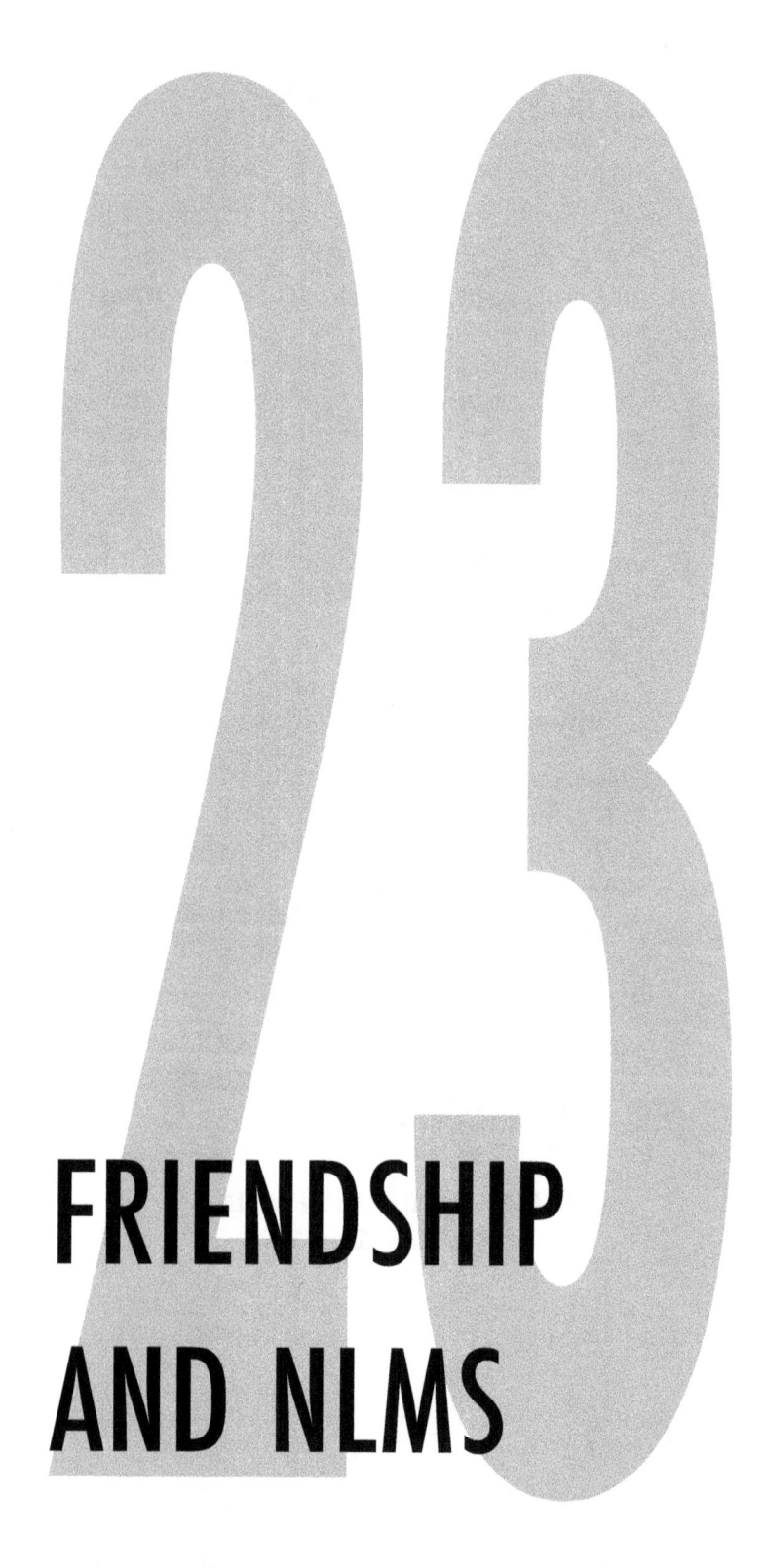

FRIENDSHIP AND NLMS

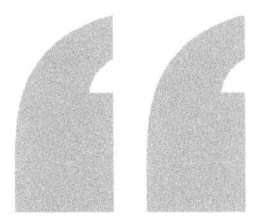

> Friendship with oneself is all important because, without it, one cannot be friends with anybody else in the world.
>
> — Eleanor Roosevelt

BOUNCER: Someone needs your friendship. Be the friend.

What a beautiful voice. As I followed the music, I found three people laughing and singing around the piano in my college union one morning when I stopped in to grab a cup of coffee. It was the first week of classes and there was a newness in the air with the excitement of meeting new friends. Everyone was embarking on a journey into the unknown... their future.

Two good-looking young guys playing guitars, a red-head they called Red Dog, and a blond I soon discovered was affectionately referred to as *Sexie Rexie*, were sitting by a piano where a young girl with the most incredible voice and engaging smile completed their trio. They were laughing and singing, filling the room with song and smiles, and capturing a growing audience. It was contagious. I was hooked as I joined the crowd. That day, I met someone who would soon be one of the best friends I had in the world. We clicked. It didn't take long for me to see that the girl with the beautiful voice also had a beautiful heart. We laughed together and acted crazy, and soon, became roommates. I never got that cup of coffee, but I got a lifelong friend.

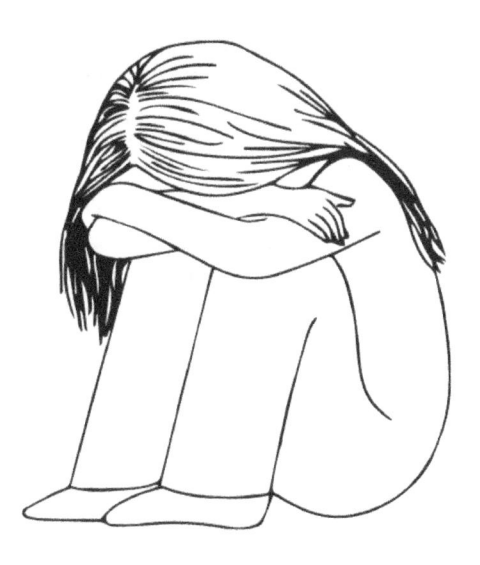

I didn't find out until many years later that as a little girl, her parents had become ostracized in their tiny community because of religious decisions they made. Consequently, the fallout labeled their only daughter an outcast in her school where other children were not allowed to play with her. None of this was her fault. She was an innocent victim of cruel and narrow-minded self-righteousness. What a loss for those whose blind ignorance made them miss an opportunity for an incredible friendship. A lesson we could learn from. It was a tragedy of misplaced judgment.

I was the first friend she ever had.

I DON'T KNOW HOW TO MAKE FRIENDS

"I watch you and you have a lot of friends." Her voice was quiet as we sat in the restaurant. "How do you make friends? I don't know how." Her pain was almost palpable.

I heard this frequently over the years as a restaurant owner, and each time, the same word came to mind. Like a bartender or hairdresser, I learned a lot about my customers and their lives while talking to them, and more importantly, listening. It didn't take long for them to open up about what was on their minds. People with problems want to talk–they need to, especially to someone who is *safe*. Whether taking care of the sick as I did in my nursing career, or feeding hungry people, I understood the importance of making people feel special instead of being just another customer. *Just another...* a lonely feeling of being lost in the crowd. So, I listened.

Remembering was important–anything about them and their lives, big or small, shouted that they belonged. "How was Sammie's soccer game?" or "Did you get that job you were interviewing for?" was like everyone in *Cheers* calling out "Norm!" when he came through the door... *where everybody knows your name.* Little personal things that I could ask about the next time I saw them made the difference in feeling they belonged. And contrary to what some may believe... that's better than okay. I can't imagine a better compliment than when customers brought in friends who said they were told it was like eating at their grandma's dinner table.

But I couldn't tell you most of their names. Were they friends?

WHAT IS FRIENDSHIP?

- The epitome of happiness. The epitome of pain.
- The epitome of fulfillment. The epitome of empty.
- The epitome of self-judgment. The epitome of misperception.

- The epitome of complicated. The epitome of simple.

A RECENT UK STUDY OF MILLIONS OF PEOPLE FOUND THAT ONE IN 10 PEOPLE FELT THEY DIDN'T HAVE A CLOSE FRIEND, AND ONE IN FIVE NEVER OR RARELY FELT LOVED.

Friends have a tremendous impact on our lives, so it makes sense that those with NLMS, who struggle with relationships and are prone to believing that nobody wants to be their friend, are severely affected. Feeling that you don't have friends, no one to call when you reach for the phone, and even worse, not knowing how to make them is terribly dispiriting. My heart went out to those who approached me in the restaurant. It's agonizing to discern that everyone else has friends but you. This is nurtured by Nagatha, of course, but know it's an illusion... not based on reality. Having realistic *expectations* of friendship is a game-changer for self-esteem and self-confidence. It was one of the worst things I battled with NLMS and must have been easily recognized by those who professed to fit into their circle of friends with ease. But that was before I understood cliques and the complicated wheels of insecurity churning within us all, camouflaged better by some than others.

I AM UNLIKABLE = I DON'T HAVE FRIENDS

I DON'T HAVE FRIENDS = MEANS NOBODY LIKES ME

We need friendship, just like we need to be liked, so why is it so hard for some? Could it be that *thinking you are unlikable* is the reason you don't have friends? Or does not having friends cause you to feel that nobody likes you? They may sound the same, but there's a difference. If you feel you are not likable, it can keep you from seeking out friends. Why bother, right? I'll only impose myself on others who don't want to be around me because they don't like me. The second scenario is the opposite, assuming the reason you don't have friends is because you are not likable, meaning that nobody has tried to be your friend. In my former state of mind, I rationalized turning up the dial on the emptiness I felt. Who would want to be friends with someone they didn't like, or more accurately, with *someone who doesn't like themselves?*

But what if... you liked yourself? I got the answer when I flipped my selfie and faced off with Nagatha. The fog lifted and my life completely turned around. I discovered that you attract positive things (like friends)... when you are just you. That's all anyone is looking for.

Getting to know what friendship is (apart from your misperceptions), and having realistic expectations (i.e., I don't need a flock, so no more clingy needy Nellie), will open your door to real friendship–opposed to assumptions. Friends will happen. They will come to you. Appear when you aren't looking. Flip your selfie... and clean out your what *I think I gotta have closet*. You may be able to spend the money on treating yourself to something a lot more fun than buying and reading books on *how to make friends*.

THE SECRET TO FRIENDSHIP

First, are you ready for friendship? Can you be 110 percent honest with who you are? Are you secure enough to put it all on the table to be a genuine friend, to let go of the fear, and not hold back? As David Essel says in his book, *Love and Relationship Secrets That Everyone Needs To Know*, "Risking who we are authentically, who we are when no one is around." Friendship is about being open and honest, trusting without fear of being judged or abandoned. It's a two-way street. It's about mutual respect.

Second, do you have time for multiple friends? A common misperception by those with (and some without) NLMS is that you have to have *a lot of friends*, like the fake groups you wrongly label on social media. The number of friends a person has depends on personalities, age, and especially lifestyle. Friends are an asset that require

friends Come in Different Shapes & Sizes

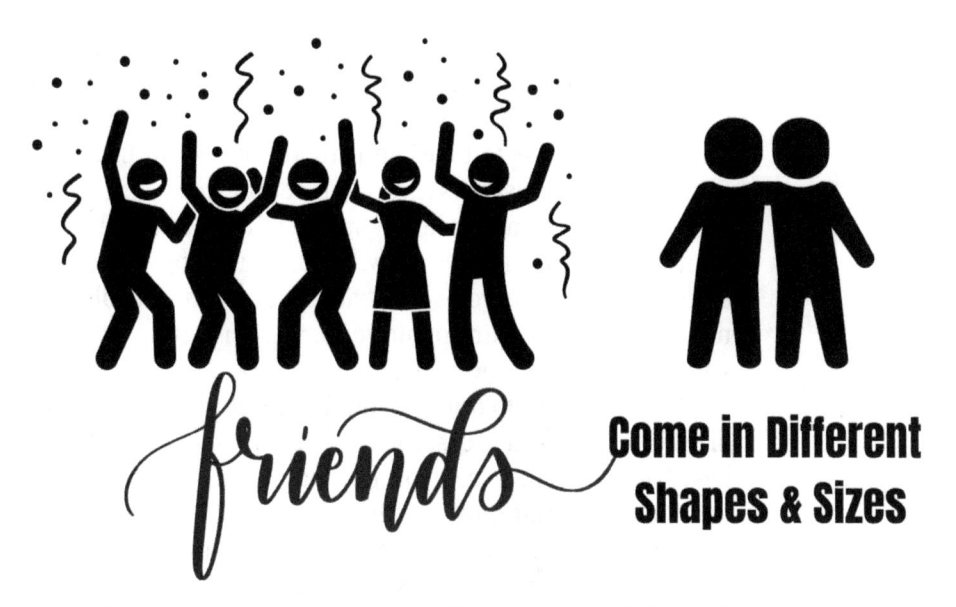

your time and energy, consequently, your schedule and commitments must be a consideration in the number of friends you can effectively manage. A single person with no children may find it easier to manage more friends than one married with the added responsibility of children. And then there is individual preference. It's not uncommon to have just one good friend by choice. Of my three kids, two ran in swarms and the other had one good friend at a time. They were all happy and content.

MISCONCEPTION

The word that came to mind each time I heard… "I watch you and you have lots of friends," was misperception–Nagatha's soul-mate. And it's rampant. Their misperception was a result of not understanding the difference between friendship and showmanship. Seeing people in friendly conversations created the illusion that everyone had friends but them. What is their misperception?

***BEING FRIENDLY WITH PEOPLE
MEANT THEY WERE YOUR FRIENDS.***

There's a difference between friendly and friend. Friendly is an adjective and simply means kind and pleasant. It has nothing to do with being a friend (which is a noun that means "to love" and "to honor" in old English). Conversely, *friendship* is a verb, an action word, a process, an art, which comes with responsibilities and commitments not to be taken lightly. Before jumping to the assumption that everyone has friends but you, disable the misperceptions, your cognitive distortions, and put what you are seeing into perspective.

It's important to understand that there are many levels of *friends;* acquaintances, casual friends, close friends, and best friends. Which are you talking about? You probably have many acquaintances, which happens just by going to the grocery store or various meetings. Good or best friends, the level most people are thinking about when they think, "I don't have friends," always *start* as acquaintances–which is what the customers in my restaurant were observing. Some of those did grow into casual or close friends over time, which is how friendships develop... over time. All of them. *Love at first sight* happens, but friendship develops.

MISREPRESENTATION

Social media–the thing you love to hate and hate to love. It is powerful when not abused–and powerful when it is. You can reach everyone in the world with a single click, making it essential for businesses to communicate and be successful in today's world. I loved it when promoting our restaurant, bringing in customers from around the world and helping us to get voted the 4th Best BBQ Restaurant in America. We certainly couldn't have been as competitive without it.

But for an 'I need friends' addict, social media is like their dope dealer when they need a fix... all too happy to be their den of misrepresentation. Disingenuous posts clearly mislead the needy who are looking for friends in all the wrong places.

Ironically, it's a two-way road of deceit when those posting are just as needy, nursing their own insecurities by fiercely posting pictures of themselves at events–surrounded by so-called friends to show the world how *popular* they are. Although they don't know most of the people in the picture, the implication can send someone who falsely feels that nobody likes them straight into a depression, oblivious to the facts–that those in the picture happened to be in the right place at the right time to be part of a cattle call... everyone, huddle in close for a picture. I've been there plenty of times and found myself feeling a little like an extra on a set... where everybody doesn't know your name.

Misrepresentations are everywhere, people desperate to be seen the way they want to be seen. On your journey, learn to see them for what they are. Allow me to get on my bandwagon about the terror and error of social media in the next chapter, Nagatha Nests.

REALISTIC EXPECTATIONS

- What do you expect from friendship?
- What do you need from friendship?
- What do you want from friendship?

Do an *expectations* check-up! Are yours realistic? Or have they been influenced by distortions of what you thought you were seeing... or maybe wanted to. Like soap operas that have one of the most detrimental effects on marriages. In my younger idealistic years, I struggled with romantic relationships that never seemed to work out. When a savvy friend gave me a book about being in love with love, like her, I finally figured out that I was in love with the fairy tale. And that fairy tale was always going to be over when I woke up to dirty undies and socks on the floor. Friendship is the same. Are you looking for the fairy tale in a friendship? If you're waiting for the perfect friend to come along who is going to fulfill all of your needs, they'll be riding in on the same horse as Prince Charming and Sleeping Beauty.

Like any relationship, friendships come, and for various reasons... they go. It's not unusual to feel rejected or take it personally when that happens. We are herd animals by nature and crave a space of belonging. Friendships fill that space and meet our emotional needs. Depending on our personalities, our stations in life and experiences, we all desire and need different things in friendships.

Some of the more common things we look for in friendship are:

- **Companionship** - Companionship lets us know that we are not alone in this crazy world we live in. And that's a great feeling. Our discomfort of isolation and being alone, yearning for deeper connections with others, and a sense of belonging are what energize us to seek out friends. Although we sometimes try to numb lonely feelings with crutches like food, TV, or indulging in the make-believe world of social media, those are only temporary solutions to the greater need for relationships. Research shows that people who are socially active, even in small ways, tend to live longer and have a decreased risk of developing depression.

- **Fun** - Fun is the fizz that comes with friendship and keeps it alive.

- **Empathy** - Empathy is the greatest superpower that meets a deep psychological need of sharing feelings and emotions with someone.

- **Assistance** - Friends help each other. Someone to call who has your back.

- **Learning** - Friends teach us life lessons like my Asian neighbor.

Most of us don't consciously think about what we want or need in a friend. We just find them in the same places we like to go, doing the same things we like to do... so we're naturally drawn to them. Because we have the same interests and values, we can fulfill each other's needs. We just connect.

There are friends and connections out there for everyone, but unrealistic goals can feed the fear of rejection. Everyone is hoping someone will reach out to them, just like you. Take the initiative and... be the friend.

Once you understand friends, what they are, how to make them, and you get your expectations lined up with reality, you're going to take the wheel and rid yourself of misguided self-pity as you enjoy the show along with your new best friend... you.

HOW DOES IT MAKE YOU FEEL WHEN YOU SEE PEOPLE WHO APPEAR TO HAVE A LOT OF FRIENDS?

Do you hear Nagatha's lying soundtrack in your head reminding you that you are

LONELY... UNWANTED... FRIENDLESS... UNLIKABLE...

BECAUSE NOBODY LIKES YOU?

Do you believe that if you don't have friends, there must be something wrong with you?

TELL NAGATHA TO PUT A SOCK IN IT

You may be wondering what happened to my friend who spent tortuous years in grade school with no friends after being unfairly ostracized. Her story is a testimonial to the importance of building that protective shield around the soft clay at birth. Because she was made to feel loved and accepted with a strong sense of belonging early on, her strong self-esteem and confidence held, and she survived, living a happy, successful life. We are still friends. What should you expect from friendship? Only what you can give. Be choosy.

FLIP YOUR SELFIE ACTIONS:

Take a look at your friendship meter. Being completely honest is the key to your progress.

1. If you feel you don't have real friends, is it because:

A. Nobody likes you?

B. You don't like yourself and alienate others by believing you don't deserve to have friends?

2. Are you making excuses? I.E., I don't know how to make friends. A lot of people do, which is why authors are making a fortune on all the books they write about how to make friends. (You won't need the others after this book.)

3. Are you projecting your feelings of being unlikable onto others, inadvertently being uninviting by putting up walls to protect yourself from rejection?

In my NLMS life, I would have answered:

1. Yes to both.

2. I had no problem trying but felt like I was a failure and doing something wrong.

3. Probably not.

Now I would answer:

1. Not anymore. I have great friends.

2. No, my expectations have changed.

3. Not anymore.

24
NAGATHA NESTS

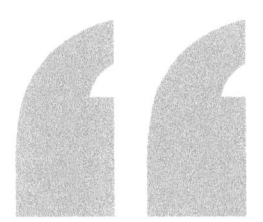

> Don't be a victim of negative self-talk. Remember, YOU are listening.
>
> -Bob Proctor

BOUNCER:

I will not allow myself to be a victim.

"That's so high school!"

Have you ever said that?

High school is the epitome of a Nagatha Nest. A place full of vulnerable young minds under construction. What comes to mind when you think back to your high school days? Gossip. Cliques. Ridicule. Not being nominated for even one queen. Like me. *Am I still obsessing over that?* Making the football team. Almost. A boyfriend stolen by a friend. Or how about being the last one chosen for... anything? If there was ever a time to get hit square in the face with "Nobody Likes Me Syndrome," it's high school, but let's just take a leap further back to grade school. These could seem like some of the roughest years of your life. Egos bouncing around from wall to wall like a bat in a cave looking for light as they search to find their way and digging out from the hormone avalanche of who you are. Some mature earlier than others, and then there are those who never get there. Self-esteem and confidence are in their infancy, vacillating from obnoxiously over-confident to none at all.

The thought of having to go back to those years and do it all over again makes me cringe. Unless I could go back, knowing what I know now. I would rule with my 20/20 hindsight vision about my former roommate, Nagatha.

ENTER AT YOUR OWN RISK

Is your shield strong enough to withstand a Nagatha Nest and come out unscathed?

Nagatha haunts can be magnets for needy people who are desperate to be accepted. They can be anywhere if there is a spotlight to be had. People with troubled self-esteem that constantly needs to be reinforced will seek out opportunities like organizations, clubs, committees, teams, nightclubs, and church leagues. Coincidentally, these places are always looking for needy people to do thankless volunteer jobs. "Club President" can be rough on friends and family but looks good on the resume. That doesn't mean there aren't very confident people who are competent leaders and enjoy leadership positions. *Put your hand down Tommy, we'll get to you.* Just be careful not to use this kind of over-involvement as the Band-Aid for lacking self-love. It can be treacherous and keep you on the downhill slope you were trying to reverse. People in this kind of nest who question their own worth can be rattlesnakes... defensive and petty, fighting among themselves for positions, and hurtful in an attempt to feel better about themselves.

WHEN WAS THE LAST TIME YOU TOOK A SELFIE?

Have you ever watched a movie with undesirables you wouldn't want to hang out with... the bad guys? The camera pans a dark, smoky room with foreboding music and characters that appear to have common goals. And they do... just not good ones. They don't want to be there, nobody does, but at least they have a place to belong (not one they want to identify with, but at least it's belonging somewhere.) Maybe in the movie they're thieves or drug dealers or alcoholics, but at least they aren't alone. *Okay, so I have a vivid imagination.* That may be a bit of a dramatization, but you get the point. Any group in a pinch isn't better than no group.

When I flipped my selfie, it was all right there in front of me, and I didn't like the movie I was watching. I didn't want to identify with desperate. I didn't want to be pathetic. It wasn't the real me, the person with self-regard I wanted to be. I didn't want to belong to organizations just for the sake of belonging somewhere. I wanted to have the courage to say no. Yes, didn't make anyone like me, it enabled myself to be used. I felt weary, like everything was wrong. It took years and many painful experiences before I crawled out enough to see the truth. The only way to be in a real spotlight is to make your own. Nagatha Nests can sink you deeper into despair.

THE ABSOLUTE WORST NAGATHA NEST

Social media! (Allow me to get my megaphone and step onto my bandstand.) It's everywhere and so easily available to everyone, any time, at the touch of a finger. It's the local bar that people clamor to, the shoulder to cry on, the hunting ground for those who prey on the vulnerable. It is used and abused. If you must use it, do so conscientiously for the right reasons. If you find it makes you feel down... stay off.

People on social media may agree with your politics, your opinion, your religion, or your vision, but most don't know you and don't necessarily want to. Surveys show that kids are one of the top five things people hate to see pictures of on social media, along with food and vacations. What else is there? People just want your 'like'! They aren't looking to connect over lunch or listen over a glass of wine to your heartaches. Likes and friends on social media are empty and meaningless! It's competition to see who has the most... a terrible misuse and abuse of the word. My Facebook page usually maintains close to the maximum (unless you're Taylor Swift) of 5,000 friends. I don't know most of them. People will say, "Aren't we friends on FB?" I don't know, are we? If they were actually a "friend", I would probably know it.

Think of much time you spend on social media and more importantly, why. Keep a log for a few days. You may be surprised. Understand where the Nagatha Nests are and decide if this is where you want to spend that time. You would get more YOU benefits face-to-face with a friend. Trade three hours of social media for a very nice one-on-one lunch. One-upmanship gets you what? If you feel the need to be a name-dropper, don't forget to change your handle to 'I'm Needy!' Or just wear a sign on your chest.

The positive side is that it is a place to share information when you lose a loved one, ask for prayers, or want to catch up with old friends. I've hooked up with long-lost relatives or classmates I've lost track of, which made me remember why. I find it especially amusing, maybe because we grow up and our priorities change, that what was life or death, worth killing for in high school, doesn't matter anymore–and how about those classmates we didn't particularly like who are now our friends? Long forgotten are the catfights and cliques we were ostracized over... what was it again? We all grow up.

Over the years, as I became more secure with who I was, I learned that Nagatha Nests are everywhere and will

> "If we do not create and control our environment, our environment creates and controls us."
>
> —Marshall Goldsmith

always exist as long as you allow yourself to be vulnerable. It took a lot of experience to wake up to, you can't be a victim... unless you give your permission.

It's your life. You are in control... of everything. Here's the remote control. Turn off the TV. Don't put on a movie you like. PRODUCE IT!

DESIGN YOUR ENVIRONMENT SO IT NOURISHES WHO YOU WANT TO BE

Create an environment for yourself that nourishes the real you and who you want to be, not someone you think others want you to be. Unlearn needing to be in the right place with the right people and be where you are with people you genuinely enjoy doing the things you like with.

DON'T FALL INTO A NAGATHA NEST BEFORE LOCKING YOUR DOOR.

FLIP YOUR SELFIE ACTIONS:

1. Write a scene in the movie of your life. Is it a movie you want to be in?

    A. If not, write a scene in the movie you want to be in.

2. Make a list of the people you hang out with and the places you go, and why. Do you genuinely enjoy them? Or do you just want to belong somewhere?

3. Describe your ideal environment you would control, including who you would have in it.

PART IV
ABOUT EVICTING NAGATHA: THE NEW YOU

I AM CONFIDENT

The woman I once was said, "You're very arrogant, aren't you?" I said, "No, I'm confident." She said, "What is the difference?" I answered, "Arrogance is overcompensating for a known weakness; confidence is knowing your strengths, but also knowing your weaknesses, enabling you to improve them."

Avoid hiding behind your strengths for fear of your weaknesses being revealed. Ironically, freely exposing your weakness is a sign of strength.

- Author Unknown

25
CONQUERING
WITH
CONFIDENCE

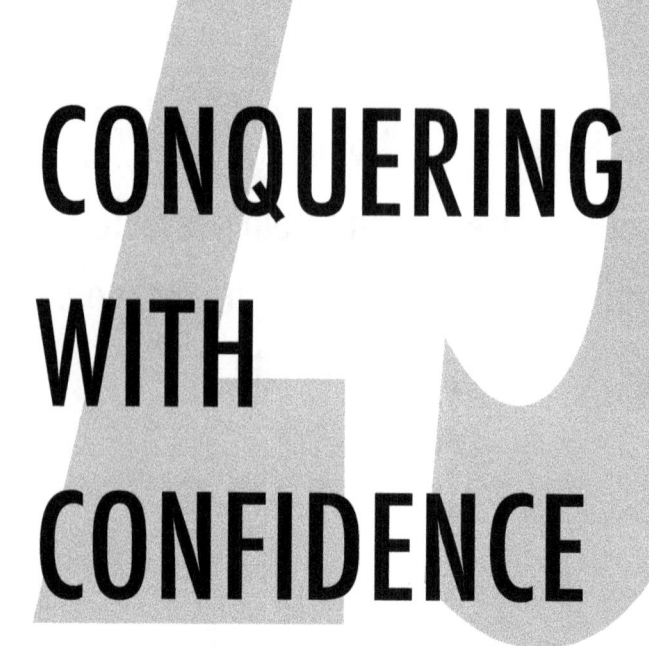

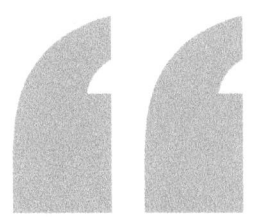

Confidence is silent.
Insecurities are loud.

- Joel Osteen

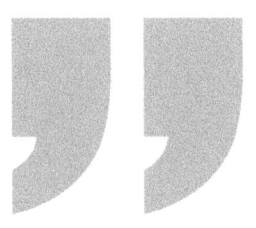

BOUNCER:
Nobody is good enough to get me down.

> Don't wait on confidence to take action.
> Self-clarity creates your confidence.
> Be present and stay in your own embodiment.
> Do you have clarity of who you want to be?

IMA WINNER

Think of yourself as a winning racehorse. We'll call you IMA WINNER. The only problem is that you rely on being liked and accepted by others to keep you going. Their approval and recognition are your feed–the bag of oats that nourishes you. You feel you need it to win. The problem is that while positive feedback is good, what happens when you don't get it? Or worse, what if it's negative? Relying on others is frustrating and... *unreliable*. It makes you needy–an addict needing a fix. When the oats run out, you start losing races. Your name becomes IMA LOSER! Not good.

The only thing about people you can count on is that *you can't count on people*. But there is one thing you can always count on–you. And only you. The *putting yourself first rule* applies to everyone. Give yourself the exclusive power and privilege to feed yourself and stop relying on other people to fuel you. Understanding what you need to win enables you to create your own recipe for your bag of oats–a formula that will nurture you with confidence and freedom. What you get from others is the gravy.

IMA WINNER FORMULA

1. BE AWARE OF YOUR STRENGTHS AND TALENTS AND BOLDLY LEAN INTO THEM.

These are potent gifts. Don't let them go unnoticed. Nothing builds your self-confidence (and self-esteem) more than accomplishments–sweeping negative thoughts about yourself out the door and ushering in positive ones. Be your own cheerleader, focusing on one positive thing a day and proudly cheering the YOU team to victory.

2. FLIP YOUR SELFIE AND MAKE YOUR LIFE ABOUT YOU.

Clearly define and write down what you want in life that will make you happy... then do it.

Do things just for you, not just for the approval of someone else. (This could include things you do for others that bring you joy.) Re-script your mind to do them WITHOUT GUILT. Eventually, your old thinking will fade away, and your new script will be strong enough to shut the door in the face of your nasty roommate. It's a happy day of wonderful *take your breath away* freedom when you look at Nagatha in the mirror and say, "*You're outta here!*"

3. GENUINELY (WITHOUT APOLOGY) LIKE YOURSELF AND BE YOUR OWN BEST FRIEND.

That means treating yourself like one. Greet yourself in the mirror every day with a hearty "Good morning!" Too much humble is overrated... and nauseating. Enjoy your own company. When you actually like yourself *for real*, you don't have to tell anyone, they'll know, and want what you have. Toss the idea that it is wrong in the garbage and take out the trash. *Like yourself and others will follow.*

4. GRACIOUSLY ACCEPT RECOGNITION AND COMPLIMENTS.

You deserve it. It puts a spring in your step and makes you feel great. Anyone who denies that is just lying. We are human. But as much as you love it and want it, you won't need it in an unhealthy way with your new formula. It's the dessert after getting your daily requirements. You will thrive beautifully on liking yourself, self-recognition, and approval.

5. FEED YOURSELF WITH POSITIVE THOUGHTS THAT MAKE YOU FEEL HAPPY AND SATISFIED.

Like the smoothie full of the healthiest nutrients I make for myself every morning, take the best care of yourself you can because you genuinely love yourself and who you are.

- It may take a while before you feel comfortable with this self-love, but don't give up.
- Start with small steps and practice.
- Retrain your mind to like you... then love you. They are not mutually exclusive.
- Laugh at yourself. Perfection can be boring.
- Create your own positive triggers about yourself to replace the former negative ones.
- Don't wait for others to praise you, it may never happen. Praise yourself for not only big things, but little things every day–little nothings that make you smile.
- Learn to say, "I am worth it," and notice the changes in the way you feel about yourself.
- Stop relying on others to make you feel good.
- Ask yourself why the opinion of others matters more than yours.
- Stop being a people-pleaser. The only person you need to please (other than your boss) is #1... YOU.
- Give people sincere recognition and compliments they deserve because you want to, not to make them like you.
- And the best part... watch for the change in the way people treat the new confident you... the one who exhibits self-love.

YOU ARE WRONG, NAGATHA

PEOPLE LIKE REAL PEOPLE WHO ARE CONFIDENT AND LOVE THEMSELVES.

SLUMPS

Everyone hits slumps, even those of us who are the happiest and most secure. Be on the lookout and recognize them for what they are–a temporary dip in the road, immediately followed by a hill that puts us back on top... if you don't lose your momentum. It's just Nagatha trying to slip in the back door to no avail because it's locked, and you are still in control. When I'm overwhelmed, I find myself more susceptible to hitting slumps, but even then, I'm armed and ready with bouncers. Learn to recognize your triggers. They can be hormones that stir-up emotions, a challenging situation, or most commonly for me, fatigue... the enemy and Nagatha's doorman. She never gives up. Fall back on your knowledge, self-love, and bouncers to shield yourself. Then throw her out. Her lies are still lies.

DAILY RENEWALS PROTECT YOU FROM FALLING INTO A SLUMP, OFTEN TAUGHT IN SELF-HELP COUNSELING.

1. *A daily morning or bedtime self-evaluation* of yourself is a strong way to start or end your day. Look at yourself in the mirror and have a power chat about your self-worth, values, and personal development. It's a powerful exercise that will reinforce your approval of yourself, keep your thoughts and mind healthy, strong and moving in the right direction, and prevent Nagatha from slipping in.

2. **Constantly talk to yourself, saying positive things** about who you are, what you do, AND what you want to be. Repeat compliments you have heard from others that gave you a boost and add a few of your own. Praise yourself out loud for accomplishments and name your positive results. I nailed that project, and everyone loved it. If you need a pep talk about something you want to achieve, become your own motivational speaker. Become a film director, creating your own personal reel of self-affirmations and then believe them. As alien as it may seem at first, it will soon become routine when you begin to believe them.

3. **Don't expect to change overnight.**

4. **Writing in a journal**, even a few thoughts a day, is a great exercise.

5. **And of course, praying is the ultimate.**

You've heard the saying garbage in, garbage out. Fill your mind with goodness. Enlightening activities like reading positive articles, supporting others with encouraging, purposeful thoughts about them, helping someone in need and listening to motivational podcasts will take out the garbage.

The healthier your mind is, the more you will:

- Like yourself
- Love yourself
- Approve of yourself
- Respect yourself
- And the happier you will be.

> Get your feet securely under you.
> Stand tall and proud of who you are.

EVEN WHEN THE SKY IS HEAVILY OVERCAST, THE SUN HASN'T DISAPPEARED, IT'S JUST HIDDEN BY DARK CLOUDS.

We are born with no preconceived thoughts about ourselves until Nagatha finds us somewhere along the way. We pick up negative feelings, learn self-criticism, self-doubt, and question our self-worth–no matter how accomplished or educated we become. She lingers within us all and affects us every day.

Science shows that up to 95 percent of what we do as adults is dictated by subconscious patterns learned when we were children. It's time to reclaim what is rightfully yours and take back your power to experience unwavering confidence. What if you could hit reset and clear your subconscious of *outdated limiting beliefs*? Imagine a life with nothing held back... a life where you are truly unstoppable.

Do you see it?

Do you see yourself grabbing the brass ring and not looking back? A life that can be yours by uncovering and replacing your deepest limiting beliefs with powerful mental frameworks of unstoppable confidence. I hung motivational posters in my kids' room. My favorite... If you can dream it, you can be it... because you can. How can you make anything happen if you can't first see it happening?

Pursue your dreams with your eye on your North Star, leaving the nay-sayers in your dust, in your wake of determination.

—Arvey

> "Can you remember who you were before the world told you who you should be?"

—Danielle LaPorte

Your mind is constantly seeking happiness while love, joy, and peace are constant states deep within you trying to GET OUT. Albeit, they are a part of you, they can be covered beneath dark clouds–negative thoughts. Until you have freed yourself of Nagatha, they can't surface and flourish.

You will never be a finished product because you have so much to offer. Aren't you glad? You will always be a work in progress... and fortunately, you are the architect, the designer. You can make your creation anything you want it to be. You can be the you that... you visualize. Get out of your own way.

Live the life you know you can attain by not self-sabotaging your success.

Reward yourself for accomplishments, big or small.

Make yourself chocolate chip cookies to say thanks to you for being you.

ME AND ME

If you were isolated from others and there was no one else around to impress, would you still try to be better? I have a running shirt I wear in the mornings for my five-mile walk that says Me vs. Me. One morning, a young guy who looked to be in high school said, "I like your shirt," as we passed on the trail. That reinforced my belief that even if it was just Me vs. Me, most of us would try to be better because we genuinely care about what we think of ourselves. It also sends a message. If there is no one else around, you are obviously doing it for the right reason. Must be love.

Every day, I like to challenge myself with small things because, collectively, they become big things. Can I repeat that recipe and make it better? Can I fold the clothes faster and more efficiently? Can I devise a way to water the plants more quickly? Little victories between me and me are fun and make me happy, whether it's tasks around the house or walking a faster mile. *Me and me* have a lot of fun together... NOW that Nagatha is gone. I still think about her once in a while and remember how miserable and needy she made me. I smile to myself. *Me and me* don't miss her.

There will always be those who didn't get the memo that we are supposed to do good things just for ourselves. Who could criticize that? Those who haven't been to Nagatha Boot Camp and still believe they shouldn't be kind to themselves. After all, they don't deserve to be happy with who they are. They even feel guilty when trying to please themselves. It's just wrong! And don't you dare say something nice about yourself. You'll be condemned for life. Should someone ask if you are good at doing something, vehemently deny it. Nobody likes a bragg-ster... hand them Nagatha.

FLIP YOUR SELFIE ACTIONS:

1. Write the recipe for your IMA WINNER feedbag.

2. We all have slumps. Track your slumps and try to identify the triggers that put you there.

3. Make a list of your daily renewals and a schedule for you to follow to use them.

4. If you could hit a reset button, what limiting beliefs would you reset?

    Get a sketch pad and draw the unstoppable life you visualize for yourself.

5. If you were isolated with no one around to impress, what would you:

    A. a. Do the same?

    B. b. Try to do better or worse?

    Now discuss why with yourself.

26
EVICTING NAGATHA

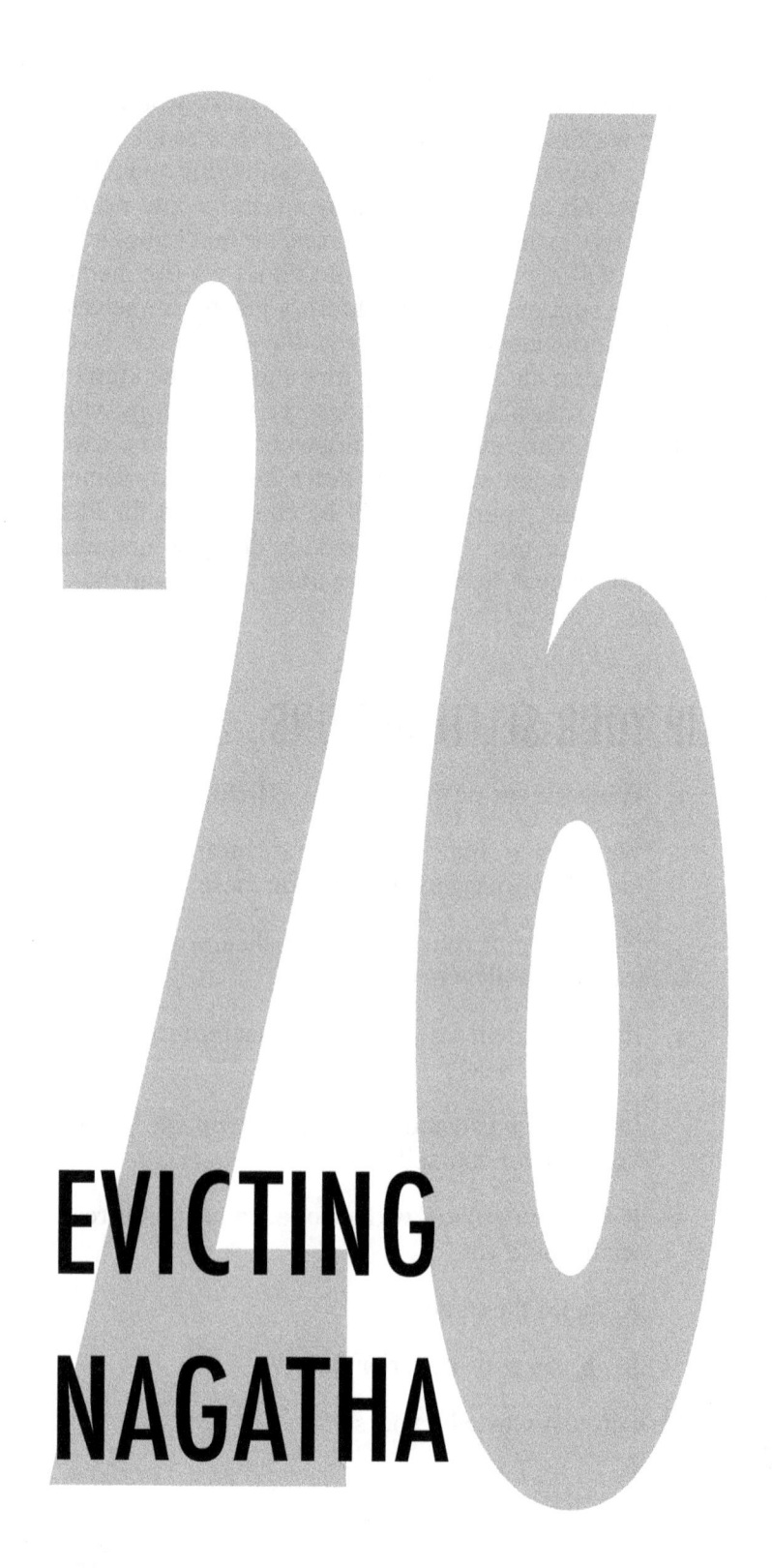

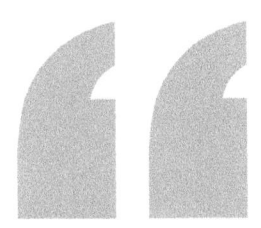

> **Being aware of this inner critic and its ability to limit you is an important part of silencing it.**
>
> - Humaira Syed, *55 Habits for Mindset Mastery: A Perfect Collection of Everyday Simple HABITS to Change Your Life Forever*

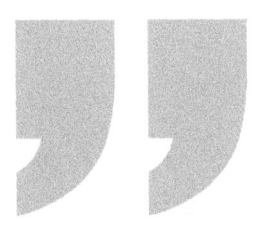

BOUNCER:
Take off your mask and be who you are—without apology.

It's the moment you've been waiting for–the end of your journey with Nagatha. It's time to say goodbye. Have you done a bed check? She may have already slipped out the back door the same way she came in.

You have been weaponized with:

- Self-confidence.

- An understanding of other people.

- Positive, wonderful knowledge about yourself you are bristling with: who you are and your undeniable self-worth.

- Recognizing the difference between want and need, and no longer feeling needy.

- Genuinely liking yourself *and* loving yourself–just the way you are.

- No longer needing the approval of everyone else because you have your own.

- The freedom of choosing who to like and who to be friends with... instead of *needing* to be chosen.

- Being guilt-free.

When you realize that the person behind the mask doesn't have to be the first one chosen and doesn't have to always be right, you have made it. You have reached a level of maturity and confidence to openly be you–mask-free.

- You are your new best friend, with a healthy mindset and perspective of others.

- You no longer assume that what others say and do is about you. It's about them. Your eyes are open wide.

- You are comfortable around others and accept that you don't need or even want to be liked by everyone. In the real world, where you now live, it's more than okay–it's good.

- You know the reasons you may like or be liked by some are the same reasons you may not like or be liked by them. You call them acquaintances and move on.

- You accept when your powerful well-managed circle is full, and your priorities are straight.

- You are real.

- Your favorite new word is... next! And it feels good.

OVERCOMING YOUR CRITICAL VOICE

Your CIV is used to being mean, and condescending, and getting away with it, but you are now trained to stop Nagatha in her tracks. The information and research pointed to in this book provides you with the weapons to stand up to these thoughts and fight back. But make no mistake... only you can use them. You are now emotionally strong, conditioned, and primed to win. One of your biggest and baddest weapons is *taking time to strategically listen to her voices with an informed knowing that... nothing she tells you is true.* Her only mission is to hurt you and secure her job. Your job is to stand up to the voices that are attacking your new friend... YOU... and use your bouncers to throw them out the door.

STEPS TO EVICT NAGATHA

A. Notice and then identify your critical inner voice–i.e., Nagatha–for what it is.

Separate it from:

- The reality of who you are.
- The world around you.
- How it alters your behavior.

B. Remind yourself where she comes from:

- Caregivers as early in your life as infancy denying you approval and validation of accomplishments (i.e., mimicking sounds and actions).
- Negative attitudes and experiences in childhood.
- Parents who suffer from their own low self-esteem and critical perceptions of themselves.
- Negative social experiences, i.e., being bullied in school, not making team sports, being embarrassed in front of the classroom by teachers, and social media (the worst culprit).

C. Write down the negative YOUs Nagatha is telling you and reword them into a bouncer.

YOU are too fat.	=	I am not fat.
YOU don't belong here.	=	I belong here.
YOU are ugly.	=	I am beautiful.
YOU are not liked.	=	I like who I am.
YOU say stupid things.	=	I say appropriate conversational things.
YOU should just shut up.	=	I fit in and am having a great conversation.
YOU are boring.	=	I am not boring.
YOU look ridiculous	=	I look good.
YOU are not making sense.	=	I am making perfect sense.
THEY are laughing at YOU.	=	They are laugh with me and having a good time.

D. When people are writing down the words of their critical voice, they may have insights that help them recognize a familiar voice or familiar words from someone in their past. Several of those I met with identify these voices as their mother or another caregiver or family member. They may identify voices they hear later in their life with someone from a former personal relationship who verbally abused them, or a teacher or boss who repeatedly belittled them for self-serving reasons. When you can recognize

> "You feel your own presence with such intensity and such joy that all thinking, all emotions, your physical body, as well as the whole external world become relatively insignificant in comparison to it."
> —A Selfless State

them, even see their faces in your mind, you will be better equipped to defeat them and kick them out.

E. Sometimes there are triggers that can cause Nagatha to rear her ugly head–possibly situations that make you feel anxious or self-conscious. A social situation with people, an event, a date, speaking engagement, or something similar may cause your self-confidence to give Nagatha a nudge and tell her it's time to go to work. Triggers are personal and will vary from person to person. They could be the result of a bad experience, like forgetting your speech while standing in a room full of people, or that hot date who never called you back. Understanding what your triggers are is not only helpful, but necessary if you are to overcome the response they evoke. To do this, journal them to help discover the correlation.

YOU ARE THE ONLY ONE WHO CAN KICK NAGATHA TO THE CURB.

Have you ever tried to convince a good friend that the guy she thinks she is madly in love with, the one you know is cheating on her, is a dirty rotten scoundrel? How did that work out for you? The longer you have lived and identified with Nagatha, allowing her to brainwash you with her lies, the deeper she is embedded in who you are, and the more you will experience resistance to evicting her. You must move into the NOW and leave the past or future. Everything is about now. People look outside for scraps of pleasure or fulfillment, for validation, for security, and for love, while they have a treasure within that not only includes all those things but is infinitely greater than anything the world can offer–something immeasurable and indestructible.

The mind is a superb instrument if used correctly. But when you allow the mind to use you instead of you using it... disease ensues. You forget who you are and believe you are your mind, the Nagathaisms. You believe the delusion and become its slave.

Your bouncers are your "OFF BUTTON". Use them to evict Nagatha... turn her off. Only then will you understand that the things that matter in your life–beauty, love, inner peace, creativity, and joy–are hidden behind the negative thoughts in the real you. Listen. Push the thoughts to the side and find yourself being present behind them. Watch and listen as they lose their power over you after being caught in the act. They will quickly subside, crawl back to where they came from when they are no longer energized by your mind identifying with them. You have empowered yourself. As this continues to happen, the frequency of Nagatha's visits will become further and further apart until they gradually disappear.

THE NEW BEGINNING OF YOU

This is the beginning of you, your natural state of feeling oneness with who you are, which has been obscured by Nagatha's disruptive thoughts. With practice, this state will deepen, and you will feel joy when you realize you like the version of you coming from deep within. In this inner connectedness, the clouds disappear, you are much more alert, and more aware of your surroundings. This state gives life to your physical body.

If you want to know your mind, the body will always give you a truthful reflection. Look at your emotion, feel it in your body. If there is a conflict, the thought will be the lie, the emotion will be the truth. It's the lie detector. It will always be reflected in the body as an emotion, and of this, you can become aware. While a thought is in your head, an emotion has a strong physical component felt in the body. You can allow it to be there without being controlled by it–you are not the emotion. If you see yourself the way your thoughts portray you, you become trapped in time, in your memories and anticipation of the future. This creates an endless preoccupation with the past. Be willing to let go and live in the present. It's difficult for some because they still see themselves in the past. They are afraid to let it go. The future is an illusion of where and what they want to be. This never brings them to now. To reality. Without letting the past and future go, you are missing the best and only reality of your life. The present.

FLIP YOUR SELFIE ACTIONS:

1. How do you feel weaponized to defeat your Nagatha?
2. Make a list of the negative YOUs you hear in your head, and your bouncer.
3. Have you done a bed check? Is Nagatha still there? Full-time, part-time, or gone?
4. Where are you living? The past, the future, or now?
5. Think about it. Have you looked behind the clouds to find your happiness hiding there? What did you find?

27
IT'S BEEN A JOURNEY

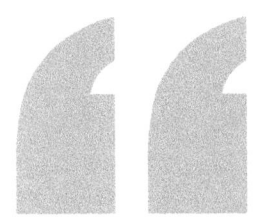

**Nobody can bring you peace
but yourself.**

- Ralph Waldo Emerson

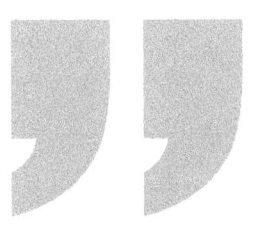

BOUNCER:

Stay the course, it's worth the trip.

My daughter and I are close. Most of the time. And most of the time is okay. We have our moments. She's probably my best friend... most of the time. At least from my vantage point as a mother. Being a teenager when she was born, we pretty much grew up together. When she got married, I carefully thought about what I wanted to say to her before she walked down the aisle... simple, but meaningful. It wasn't time for an emotional speech. It was the most anticipated day in her life, and a happy but bittersweet one in mine. After 31 years of her being the center of my world, it was time to let go and hand her over to her new husband. Before nudging her out of the nest onto the path of her fairy tale walk, I simply repeated what I had said to her so many times before, "We grew up together, and I learned so much from you. You've been a wonderful daughter, and you'll be a wonderful wife and mother. You were a gift from God, and I couldn't be prouder of the woman you are today." With a hug, a tear, and a peck on her beautiful cheek, she was off to live up to those words.

My daughter and I went to the same high school in the small town we both grew up in–the kind of town where everyone knows it's 2:50 in the afternoon and there goes old Joe to the bank. Everyone knows everything about everybody. A town where you cross the street when you see your preacher, Reverend D, coming toward you on the sidewalk because you are sure he knows what you did on Friday night... along with the whole town of 10,000. How could they not? A while back, my daughter said someone (the mothers of her friends and I were classmates, so they knew everything... almost... about me) told her I was popular in high school. What? I was sure she was thinking of someone else because I never thought of myself as being popular. Sure, I was the head majorette, and a cheerleader (which was simply a popularity contest–I couldn't do so much as a somersault), but popular? That's not possible. I dated a star football player, which, in a small town, is better than being the mayor, but even with that, I was never nominated for one queen! Not one in four years. The day of the nominations, I wore the cutest outfit in my closet, smiled, and feigned surprise when someone announced it was the day to choose prom queen candidates, then anxiously watched as hands went up and names were offered. Nothing! I felt like I had been slapped in the face as I hugged the nominees and congratulated them while fighting back tears. Why not me? I had bent over backwards trying to make people like me. Joining clubs I didn't care about, laughing at terrible jokes, complimenting people on things I hated. Maybe they were just jealous. That had to be it. Years later, I laughed, probably like many others, when I read in *The Sweet Potato Queen's Book of Love* by Jill Conner Browne that she always wanted to be queen of something. Maybe I wasn't the only girl who wanted to be the queen and was never chosen. It just seemed like it at the time.

I remember the suffocating feeling of *Nobody Likes Me* as far back as grade school, even dreading going to school every day. Memories of desperately trying to make everyone like me, doing things that challenged my self-respect and intensified my self-loathing still haunt me. What I know now is that my behavior was only making it worse. But liking yourself was strictly forbidden in the world I grew up in, and self-esteem hadn't yet been discovered. How many movies have been made about troubled kids feeling like they didn't fit in and weren't liked by other kids? That was me. I may not have been the queen, but at least I was the star of something.

Popular would have never been a word I used to describe myself. I mean, not one queen nomination... forehead slap... eye roll! Seeing yourself the way others see you is hard for anybody. It's like smelling your own breath. Admit it–you have cupped your hand over your mouth and nose to try and find out what your breath smells like, too. Or maybe I'm the only weirdo here. Our opinions of others are formed through personal filters created by our individual "judgment thermometers", which doesn't make them right or wrong. They are just ours.

These schemas we form are the result of events and experiences that left their mark along the journey of our life and affect the way we see and judge ourselves... as well as others. Some are deeply buried and can be so profound that they follow us into adulthood. An example is the time I overheard my dad talking about me to my mom. He said, "I love her, but I don't like her." I was crushed–devastated.

My own father didn't like me. I quietly walked away. I never confronted him about it but have always lived with the pain of that moment. Just writing this makes me sad. If my own dad didn't like me, why would anyone else? Now that I'm older and wiser and have been on the other side, I'm sure it was a case of *smart-mouth adolescent with the shaky self-esteem of a teenager, meets the, I'm going to kill her if she doesn't grow out of this stage soon* parent.

I've been direct my whole life, and have always felt that others deserved my opinion. When someone did something to make me angry, I was proud and boastful about *putting them in their place*... meaning their place was probably no longer on my list of friends. I thought it was a badge of honor because that was the environment I was raised in–what I saw as normal behavior. Stand your ground. That was the way I saw myself. But how did others see me?

Years later, a family friend (relatively new to town) told me he had heard from people that I had a temper. I was stunned. Spirited, unafraid to go after what I wanted, but a temper? That man did me a favor that day. He opened my eyes and caused me to look at the me others were seeing. Maybe that was why I was never nominated for a queen? And it was high school as in rough crowd, "unforgiving high school". I owed him a thank you. For the first time, I saw it for what it was–a defense mechanism of someone who didn't love herself... or even like herself.

I didn't know about Nagatha then...
or that she lived in the apartment upstairs...
but the evidence is clear... she did.

DON'T BE AFRAID TO TAKE A HARD LOOK AT YOURSELF ON YOUR JOURNEY.

AS THEY SAY, YOU CAN'T FIX IT IF YOU DON'T KNOW IT'S BROKEN.

Through a lot of trials and tribulations, a lot of successes and failures in my life, I have learned to like myself–and even love myself:
Without guilt...
Without shame.

It's been a journey, painful at times, and although there will always be moments when I have to call on one of my bouncers, I made it. It's been worth the trip. You can make it too.

I AM VERY HAPPY AND PEACEFUL

What I love and value most about the new me is the peace I have inside. I no longer think about needing to make friends. I find that by just being me and loving who I am, the confidence and genuine happiness I radiate attracts friends I love who have the same values. It's like sitting by a peaceful stream where the refreshing water just keeps on flowing. I can't remember the last time I laid awake worrying about something I did or said to alienate someone. I think about the joy I feel inside. I don't worry that someone didn't text me back or ask me to have lunch. I know they will when they have time... or I ask them. By flipping my selfie, I had a startling revelation. Everything isn't about me. In fact, nothing out there is. The only thing about us is what's going on in our own lives. Isn't that wonderful?

FLIP YOUR SELFIE ACTIONS:

1. Take a trip down memory lane and think about how you felt about yourself in grade school and high school. Did you like yourself and who you were?

2. When do you remember caring about what others thought about you?

28
HAPPY RETIREMENT, NAGATHA
PUTTING THE OLD NAG OUT TO PASTURE

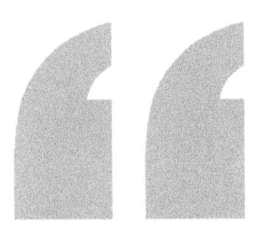

I belong deeply to myself.

- Warson Shire

BOUNCER:
I belong.

Now that you have the tools, you can build your own world, one that makes you emotionally healthy and happy. A world you control, where you choose and make confident decisions for yourself based on what you think, not what others think.

I spent, or rather wasted much of my life living with "Nobody Likes Me Syndrome." It was hard and painful, but I was the only one who knew about the monster living inside of me. You certainly don't tell others that nobody likes you, or that it's as obvious to you as everyone else that you don't belong. You suck it up. You fake it, hoping this time will be different and you will click, feeling like one of them. You long for opportunities to try again, just one more time, hoping that this time it will be different, that it will be without the voices–the relentless voices of Nagatha.

Living with NLMS is a thief that robs you of time, joy, creativity, and peace. It blinds you to realistic expectations. When I took a different road on my journey, the path of discovery and enlightenment that freed me gave me the courage to open my eyes. I also received the knowledge and awareness to flip my selfie, and to finally see reality. My quest has taken me on a long journey, but I made it, and you can too. We aren't intended to live in fear and isolation, feeling unlovable and unworthy of being liked. You have a mountain of untapped resources inside you, and uncovering them starts with your desire to let go of the fear that's been holding you back. I know you will find your freedom and the happiness you never thought possible when you evict your demons, your Nagatha, and fall in love with you and your own voice. The voice of truth... yeah, that one. The one that loves you.

> "Your heart knows if you are not where you need to be. Now your head needs to know as well. Move yourself to the number one spot on your to-do list and do what is best for you, your self-esteem, and your happiness. What a team!"
>
> —Arvey

NO MORE abusing yourself.

Now that you love yourself, you know how insane it is to abuse your best friend, the one you spend all your time with. You. Abuse is bad and you are good.

NO MORE not believing how great you are.

What's not to love? Now that your eyes are opened, celebrate the amazing you!

NO MORE not grasping your power.

You have as much power in your world as you want to have. Have the courage to use it to be happy.

NO MORE criticizing yourself.

Don't criticize... fix what you don't like and accept what you can't change. Laugh at your mistakes and take joy in being alive.

NO MORE comparing yourself to others who can't compete with you.

Flip the selfie. Do you know how many people would love to be like you? And why not? If there's something you admire about someone else, tell them. Be thankful for your own talents and style. Celebrate who you are and your uniqueness.

NO MORE judging yourself.

For what? Be thankful for the amazing person you are... your own kind of perfect. See above.

NO MORE searching for happiness.

Let it happen every day. You won't get this day back. Nobody is going to drop off a beautifully wrapped gift of perfect at your door. You already have one.

NO MORE wasting time waiting for hard times to end before you can be happy.

Chose happiness today. If you wait for hard times to end to be happy–it's not going to happen.

NO MORE caring what people think about you when they don't care what you think.

You may be the flavor of the day, but tomorrow, the menu changes.

START making the choice every morning to be happy.

You make choices from the minute you open your eyes. Make your first choice to thank God and love your day.

START pampering yourself.

Love yourself and treat you like you would anyone you love. Nah... better.

START giving yourself permission to love yourself even with the flaws you believe you have.

Thank God for your flaws and the luxury of loving you in spite of them. Perfect is overrated.

START looking at yourself and others for inspiration.

We can all be inspired by others, but don't forget all the wonderful things you have to offer.

START focusing on your strengths.

Where do you start? You have so many.

START laughing at yourself more.

Some of the funniest things in your life will be your silly mistakes. Enjoy your humanness.

START enjoying your own company.

Take yourself to dinner with a new date or a good book.

START looking at others for what they are.

This will change your life and the way you live, your perceptions, and your self-love.

START being amused at the insecurities of others.

The amusing part is the show. Hand them a copy of Nagatha and tell them they can thank you later.

FLIP YOUR SELFIE ACTIONS:

1. Start living all of the above by flipping your selfie to where your life is–you.

29
FINALE
DINNER WITH A FRIEND

It's a beautiful day.
Sun is shining.
Not a cloud in the sky.
You're wearing your shades and your favorite Saturday beach shirt.

Life is good.

A nice breeze is blowing through your rolled-down window as you drive–crooning along to the oldies with the radio. The big grin on your face pairs with the smile in your heart. Destination... wherever you decide you want to go. Maybe a movie? No, too pretty outside. The antique show in the park or a nice run along the beach? There's a great seafood festival and a live band. A crab cake sandwich from the famous Crabby Cooking food truck sounds inviting. You laugh to yourself and say out loud, "Oh, so much to do, so little time." You decide to just go where this great day takes you–follow your happy heart. This is your day.

The Crabby Cooking Crab Cake was delicious as promised, the band made you feel like a kid again, and you're heading home for a hot shower and a couple of hours of reading that novel you can't wait to finish to see if Colby finds his way to Aubry. A little later, you'll get a little dressed up to try the new restaurant in town. You've heard from friends that they have a fabulous menu, including an affordable wine list and a fun, relaxing guitarist. You're thinking the Wellington or Veal Marsala sound tasty after your very favorite appetizer, Oysters Rockefeller.

Your phone rings and it's an old friend from college inviting you to get together this evening with a group of people you've known for a long time to shoot some pool. Sounds like fun, but you can't make it.

You thank them for thinking of you and say you'll have to take a rain check.

YES. TODAY IS THE DAY. YOUR DAY.

YOU'RE HAVING DINNER WITH YOUR NEW BEST FRIEND. YOU.

30 BOUNCERS

Your bouncers are different than mine, therefore, what works for me won't always work for you. Keep your bouncers in your proverbial pocket. Even the new safe and secure you will have moments that present themselves where you may need to reach into that pocket. Spending a few minutes writing your bouncers is also an opportunity to do a self-tune-up. As new challenges evolve from incidents you encounter throughout your life, new ones will be generated. *Yes, this is normal.* Add them to your list of bouncers. You can never have too many in your arsenal.

The bouncers you have seen in this book:

1. I'm not alone, many others feel this way.
2. You are not a part of me. Why are you here?
3. Being successful, being happy, and believing in myself are the choices only I can make.
4. Be your own North Star, the only one that matters.
5. It takes grace to remain kind when people are cruel.
6. I am the director and producer of my own show.
7. You don't freely give time or space... you are robbing it from someplace else.
8. My brain is a personal computer I can reprogram.
9. Everyone isn't going to like me and that's okay.
10. Do I really like them?
11. Define normal.
12. I'm going to treat me like I love me... because I do.
13. Who are you to judge me?
14. Is that you or your ego?
15. Live up to your own expectations.
16. Lonely is an emotion–not a condition.
17. Find your wings and take flight. Connect.
18. Someone needs your friendship. Be the friend.
19. I will not allow myself to be a victim.
20. Nobody is good enough to get me down.
21. Take off your mask and be who you are–without apology.
22. Stay the course, it's worth the trip.
23. I belong.

MY BOUNCERS

NOTES

CHAPTER 2 YOU ARE NOT ALONE

1. PsychAlive, "I Hate Myself: Why Self-Hatred Occurs and How to Stop It," December 22, 2020, https://www.psychalive.org/i-hate-myself

CHAPTER 7 YOUR GATEKEEPERS

1. Rafe Ronning, (Quote) "What Are the Odds," by Mike Lindell Page 243

CHAPTER 9 PEOPLE ARE COMPLICATED

1. Zig Ziglar, *See You at The Top*, first published 1974, Crescendo Publication, Dallas. Found at most bookstores.

CHAPTER 12 THE POWER OF YOUR CRITICAL INNER VOICE

1. Madina, "The Biggest War of Life Resides Within Us... And it is only WE, who can save US from OURSELVES!" *Lines from Insane Heart*

2. Jay Earley, PhD (American computer scientist and psychologist working with the inner critic), "The Seven Types of Inner Critics", IFA Growth Programs, 2022

3. Bonnie Weiss, Psychotherapist, "The Seven types of Inner Critics", IFS Growth Programs, 2022

CHAPTER 13 YOUR POWERFUL CIRCLE

1. Ofei, Michael. "North Star What's Your North Star?" *Minimalist Vegan*. October 27, 2016. Updated June 18, 2021. Http://theminimalistvegan.com/north-star/

2. McKeown, Greg, *Essentialist*, United Kingdom: Virgin Books, 2014

3. Christie Sawyer, (Quote) "Bitterness, you have to go ..." *Arise My Love*, 2019, Christy Sawyer

CHAPTER 14 YOU CAN CHANGE YOUR BRAIN

1. Dr. Daniel Amen, "Change Your Brain change Your Life, (Lack of Focus, Anger, and Memory Problems), *Harmony*; November 3, 2015, 109-113, 149-50, 151, 105

2. Kristina Robb-Dover, "How Negative Emotions Affect Health", *FHE HEALTH*, The Florida Health Experience, June 12, 2020

3. Amy Morin, LCSW, "How to Train Yourself to Think Differently and Permanently Rewire Your Brain, According to Science - It's not about thinking positively. It's about learning how to think realistically," *INC.*, September 26, 2017

4. "It's not about thinking positively. It's about learning how to think realistically." *INC* (September 26, 2017)

5. Dr. Jeffery Schwartz (neuropsychiatrist), *Brainlock: Free Yourself from Obsessive-Compulsive Behavior*, Harper Perennial, 1997

CHAPTER 15 I JUST WANT TO BE ONE OF THE GUYS

1. Jim Kozubek, "What is Normal," Anyway?", *Scientific American*, February 22, 2018

CHAPTER 16 WHY DO I NEED TO BE LIKED

1. Roger Covid, Ph.D (Clinical psychologist,) *The Need to be Liked*, self, May 2011

2. Laura Entis, "Chronic Loneliness Is a Modern-Day Epidemic," *Fortune*, March 22, 2017(Quote from John Cacioppo (neuroscientist)

CHAPTER 17 IT'S OKAY TO NOT BE LIKED

1. James Altucher, *Choose Yourself: be Happy, Make Millions, Live the Dream*, Lioncrest Publishing, May 31, 2013

2. Dr. Ben Michaelis, Ph.D., "If Everybody Likes You, You are Doing it Wrong," *Huffpost*, April 22, 2013

3. Kurt Smith, Psy.D, LMFT, LPCC, AFC, "Is Being 'Too Nice' A Bad Thing?", *Conscious Vibe, Self-Awareness*, July 18,2022

4. Ilene Strauss Cohen, Ph.D., "How to Let Go of The Need to Please", January 25, 2021, https://doctorilene.com/2021/01/how-to-let-go-of-the-need-to-please/

CHAPTER 18 LOVING YOURSELF ISN'T GOOD IT'S GREAT

1. *The Shawshank Redemption* (Movie), Directed by Frank Darabont, USA Castle Rock Entertainment, 1994

CHAPTER 22 WHY DO I FEEL LONELY

1. John Cacioppo (neuroscientist), "Loneliness is like an iceberg... ", *The Guardian*, February 28, 2016

2. Cigna 2018 "Loneliness Index," Douglas Nemecek, M.D., MBA Chief Medical Officer for Behavioral Health, Cigna, PowerPoint Presentation (cigna.com), Microsoft Word - Loneliness_Index_National_Report_Compliance_043018_5PM.docx (multivu.com), May 2018

3. Dr. Dilip Jest, (Professor of Psychiatry and Neurosciences, University of CA, San Diego, Director of UC San Diego's Centre for Healthy Ageing),"Loneliness peaks in the 20s, 50s and 80s: US study", thejakartapost.comhttps://www.thejakartapost.com/life/2018/12/19/loneliness-peaks-in-the-20s-50s-and-80s-us-study.html, December 19, 2018

CHAPTER 23 ISOLATION IS NAGATHA

1. "Understanding the Stress Response, Staying Healthy", Harvard Health Publishing, July 6, 2020

CHAPTER 24 FRIENDSHIP AND NLMS

1. Multiple Authors *PsychAlive*, "Nobody Likes Me: Understanding Loneliness and Self-Shame", *PsychAlive*, "No-

body Likes Me:" Understanding Loneliness and Self-shame - *PsychAlive*

2. Davd Essel, M.S., O.M., *Love and Relationship Secrets... that everyone needs to know!* Gray Dog Press, 2020 Introduction